In Situ Hybridization
Principles and Practice

In Situ Hybridization

Principles and Practice

Second edition

Edited by

JULIA M. POLAK

Department of Histochemistry,
Imperial College School of Medicine, London

and

JAMES O'D. MCGEE

Nuffield Department of Pathology and Bacteriology,
University of Oxford, Oxford

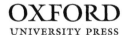

OXFORD
UNIVERSITY PRESS

This book has been printed digitally in order to ensure its continuing availability

OXFORD
UNIVERSITY PRESS

Great Clarendon Street, Oxford OX2 6DP

Oxford University Press is a department of the University of Oxford.
It furthers the University's objective of excellence in research, scholarship,
and education by publishing worldwide in

Oxford New York

Auckland Bangkok Buenos Aires Cape Town Chennai
Dar es Salaam Delhi Hong Kong Istanbul Karachi Kolkata
Kuala Lumpur Madrid Melbourne Mexico City Mumbai Nairobi
São Paulo Shanghai Singapore Taipei Tokyo Toronto
with an associated company in Berlin

Published in the United States
by Oxford University Press Inc., New York

First edition published 1990
Reprinted 1991
Second edition published 1998
Reprinted 2002

A catalogue record for this book is available from the British Library

Library of Congress Cataloging in Publication Data
In situ hybridization : principles and practice / edited by Julia M.
Polak and James O'D. McGee.—2nd ed.
p. cm.
1. In situ hybridization. I. Polak, Julia M. II. McGee, J. O'D.
(James O'Donnell)
QH452.8.I535 1998 572.894--dc21 98-39953

ISBN 0-19-854880-X

Preface to the second edition

It has given us great pleasure to see the second edition of this book reach completion.

Much has happened since the publication of our first edition and the decision to have a second one. The interest in, and application of, *in situ* hybridization have grown at an unprecedented pace and, in spite of the many difficulties that still exist, the technique(s) has matured and is used in a large number of different laboratories. In cell biology, and in pathology in particular, *in situ* hybridization has proven to be a good adjunct both for research and diagnostic purposes.

Much has happened. . . . In the midst of the preparations for this second edition, Professor Polak fell seriously ill and this delayed immensely the publication of the book. We are particularly grateful to all the contributors, who are now friends for life, for their patience and understanding. They needed to update their superb contributions several times. We are fully aware how extremely committed they all are, but they undertook their task with great understanding. Thank you all!

London and Oxford   J. M. P.
September, 1998   J. O'D. McG.

Preface to the first edition

'If there be fuel prepared, it is hard to tell whence the spark shall come that shall set it on fire'. Francis Bacon, '*Of seditions and troubles*'. Essays (1625).

Pathology is undergoing a revolution, with the arrival of new imaging methods for revealing the basic mechanisms of disease. Data provided by immunocyto-chemistry and electron microscopy are now being complemented by molecular biology. One of these techniques, *in situ* hybridization, visualizes in intact cells the genes and mRNA involved in protein synthesis. There were many difficulties to overcome in working out the methodology, but the technique is now established in many research, and some clinical laboratories. It has been rapidly adopted by pathologists and biologists.

This book forms part of a series on the practical aspects of technology at the forefront of pathology: it deals with *in situ* hybridization and its applications to the study of mechanisms underlying cellular function and disease. The authors who have contributed to this book are recognized experts and their chapters cover all aspects of *in situ* hybridization from the basic principles of molecular biology through the various methodological advances to the most up-to-date applications in developmental biology, virology, cytogenetics, and patho-biology. There is currently more emphasis on DNA than on mRNA techniques and their applications. This imbalance will be corrected with improved methodology for investigations on mRNAs in health and disease.

We are grateful to Oxford University Press for asking us to put together in a single publication these expositions of the state of the art, and latest advances, in this intriguing and fascinating laboratory technique.

'Great cultural changes begin in affectation and end in routine'. Jacques Barzan, *The house of intellect* (1959).

London and Oxford   J. M. P.
September 1989   J. O'D. McG.

Contents

Contributors

JANE ALDRIDGE
Seescan plc, Cambridge, UK

CHRISTOPHER J. BAKKENIST
University of Oxford, Nuffield Department of Pathology and Bacteriology, John Radcliffe Hospital, Oxford OX3 9DU, UK

ANTHONY P. DAVENPORT
Clinical Pharmocology Unit University of Cambridge, Addenbrookes Hospital, Cambridge CB2 2QQ, UK

KENNETH A. FLEMING
University of Oxford, Nuffield Department of Pathology and Bacteriology, John Radcliffe Hospital, Oxford OX3 9DU, UK

L. GORDON
Department of Histochemistry, Imperial College School of Medicine, Hammersmith Hospital, Du Cane Road, London W12 0NN, UK

GERARD W. HACKER
Institute of Pathological Anatomy, Immunohistochemistry and Biochemistry Unit, Salzburg General Hospital, Muellner Hauptstr. 48, 5020, Salzburg, Austria and Medical Research Coordination Center, University of Salzburg, Salzburg, Austria

C. S. HERRINGTON
Department of Pathology, University of Liverpool, PO Box 147, Liverpool, L69 3BX UK

HEINZ HÖFLER
Institute of Pathology, Technical University of Munich, School of Medicine, Ismaningstrasse 22, 81675 Munich, Germany

ANTON H. N. HOPMAN
Department of Molecular Cell Biology & Genetics, University of Limburg, PO Box 616, 6200 MD Maastricht, The Netherlands

JAMES O'D. McGEE
University of Oxford, Nuffield Department of Pathology and Bacteriology, John Radcliffe Hospital, Oxford OX3 9DU, UK

ADRIENNE L. MOREY
Division of Anatomical Pathology, St Vincent's Hospital, Sydney, Australia

Contributors

JAMES MUELLER
Institute of Pathology, Technical University of Munich, School of Medicine, Ismaningstrasse 22, 81675 Munich, Germany

J. M. POLAK
Department of Histochemistry, Imperial College School of Medicine, Hammersmith Hospital, Du Cane Road, London W12 0NN, UK

FRANS C. S. RAMAEKERS
Department of Molecular Cell Biology & Genetics, University of Limburg, PO Box 616, 6200 MD Maastricht, The Netherlands

ERNST J. M. SPEEL
Academic Hospital Nijmegen, University of Nijmegen, PO Box 9101, 6500 HB Nijmegen, The Netherlands

J. H. STEEL
Histopathology Unit, Imperial Cancer Research Fund, Room 336, 44 Lincolns Inn Fields, London WC2A 3PX, UK

MARY E. SUNDAY
Harvard Medical School and Brigham & Women's Hospital, 75 Francis Street, Boston, MA 02115, USA

RAYMOND TUBBS
Department of Clinical Pathology, Cleveland Clinic Foundation, Cleveland, Ohio, USA

PETER G. VOOIJS
Academic Hospital Nijmegen, University of Nijmegen, PO Box 9101, 6500 HB Nijmegen, The Netherlands

CHRISTINA E. M. VOORTER
Department of Molecular Cell Biology & Genetics, University of Limburg, PO Box 616, 6200 MD Maastricht, The Netherlands

MARTIN WERNER
Institute of Pathology, Technical University of Munich, School of Medicine, Ismaningstrasse 22, 81675 Munich, Germany

INGEBORG ZEHBE
Angewandte Tumorvirologie, Deutsches Krebsforschungszentrum (DKFZ), Heidelberg, Germany

Abbreviations

AAF	Acetylaminofluorene
AMCA	Amino-methyl-coumarin acetic acid
AMG	autometallography
AMV	avian myeloblastosis virus
APES	3-aminopropyltriethoxysilane
BCIP	5-bromo-4-chloro-3-indolyl phosphate
BSA	bovine serum albumin
CARD	catalysed reporter deposition
CCD	charge coupled device
CGH	comparative genomic ISH
CISS	chromosome *in situ* suppression
CML	chronic myeloid leukaemia
CMV	cytomagelovirus
CNS	central nervous system
cRNA	complementary RNA
DAB	daminobenzidine
DAPI	4, 6-diamidino-2-phenylindone
DEPC	diethyl pyrocarbonate
DMS	double minutes
DNP	dinitrophenol
DOP	degenerate oligonucleotide primed
dpm	disintegrations per minute
dsDNA	double-stranded DNA
DTT	dithiothreitol
EBV	Epstein–Barr virus
EDTA	ethylenediamminetetraacetic acid
FCM	flow cytometry
FISH	fluorescence ISH
FITC	fluoroscein isothiocynate
HPV	human papillomavirus
HSR	homogeneous staining region
HSV	herpes simplex virus
IGSS	immunogold–silver staining
ISH	*in situ* hybridization
kb	kilobase pair
LOH	loss of heterozygosity
mRNA	messenger RNA
NBT	nitroblue tetrazolium
NISH	non-isotopic ISH
NPY	neutopeptide tyrosine

PBS	phosphate-buffered saline
PCR	polymerase chain reaction
PRINS	oligonucleotide-primed ISH
PVP	polyvinylpyrrolidone
RFLP	restriction fragment length polymorphism
RT-PCR	reverse transcriptase PCR
SDS	sodium dodecyl sulfate
SSC	standard saline citrate
SSCP	single-strand conformational polymorphism
ssDNA	single-stranded DNA
SSPE	subacute sclerosing panencephalitis
ssRNA	single-stranded RNA
TdT	terminal deoxynucleotidyl transferase
TRITC	tetrarhodamine isothiocyanite
TSA	tyramide signal amplification
TSH	thyroid-stimulating hormone
YAC	yeast-activated chromosome

1

Principles of *in situ* hybridization

HEINZ HÖFLER, JAMES MUELLER, and MARTIN WERNER

Introduction

Over the past few years methods employing immunological and molecular biological techniques have had an increasingly important impact on pathology. The introduction of immunohistochemistry and Western blotting as research and diagnostic tools began a new era in pathology and led to a much clearer understanding of cell and tumour biology. Over the past decade the amount of information available through molecular biology has expanded dramatically with the development of recombinant DNA techniques, the polymerase chain reaction (PCR) and sensitive methods for the detection of specific DNA and RNA sequences by molecular hybridization. Generally, hybridization can be performed on solid supports, in solution (*in vitro*) or on tissue sections or cell preparations (*in situ*). Traditional hybridization techniques for solid supports involve the transfer of extracted and electrophoretically separated DNA fragments on to a filter (nitrocellulose or nylon membranes) followed by hybridization with a specific DNA probe (Southern blotting). Similarly, different classes of RNA isolated from a particular cell population or tissue can be identified after separation by electrophoresis and transfer on to a solid support prior to hybridization (Northern blotting). If specific DNA or RNA sequences are to be quantified without regard to their length, dot (slot) blot analysis enables rapid processing of more than a hundred samples on a single membrane. Over the past 10 years, the classical methods of Southern and Northern blotting have been increasingly superseded by DNA amplification by PCR and RNA amplification by reverse transcriptase PCR (RT-PCR), followed by detection using single strand conformational polymorphism (SSCP) and/or gel hybridization. Aside from solid supports, specific DNA or RNA hybridization can also be performed in solution in agarose gels or in microcentrifuge tubes. These techniques do not require DNA or RNA transfer on to filters and will therefore be more frequently used in the future.

Although molecular hybridization *in vitro* or to membrane-bound nucleic acids isolated from a particular cell population or tissue allows the identification of specific sequences of DNA or RNA, one learns little about the distribution of these sequences in individual cells or tissues. *In situ* hybridization (ISH), also referred as hybridization histochemistry or cytological hybridization, is a technique that, in contrast to the other methods, enables the morphological demonstration of specific DNA or RNA sequences in individual cells, tissue sections, single cells, or chromosome preparations. Hence, ISH is the only method that allows one to localize DNA and RNA sequences in a heterogeneous cell population, and thereby to determine if a gene is expressed in low levels in all of the cells or in high levels in only a few of the cells. ISH was introduced in 1969 (Buongiorno-Nardelli and Amaldi 1969; Gall and Pardue 1969; John *et al.* 1969) and was first used primarily for the localization of cellular DNA sequences. Since that time, ISH has been applied to the localization of viral DNA sequences, mRNA, and chromosomal regions. Today, ISH is one of the most powerful research tools available to the pathologist and cell biologist. In many laboratories ISH is a routine procedure, particularly for the diagnosis of viral diseases. Owing to the rapidly growing number of cloned nucleotide sequences, the number of potentially useful probes for ISH for a variety of applications is expanding quickly. Because of its high specificity and its increasing number of applications, ISH will become increasingly important in several areas of biomedical research, including developmental and cell biology, genetics, and pathology (Höfler 1987; Wolfe and Herrington 1997; Biffo *et al.* 1992).

Theoretical background of *in situ* hybridization

ISH is based on the fact that labelled, single-stranded fragments of DNA or RNA containing complementary sequences (probes) hybridize to target DNA or RNA under appropriate conditions to form stable hybrids which can then be visualized with a detection system (Fig. 1.1). Since ISH is a morphological application of primarily molecular biological techniques, the original protocols for ISH were developed by laboratories in the fields of virology and endocrinology in which recombinant DNA technology had already had a considerable impact on research activities. The optimal conditions for hybridization to purified DNA or RNA extracts on solid supports have been extensively studied and are now well described. Hybridization conditions for ISH are complicated by the fact that, in tissue sections or cell preparations, there are several factors that can lead to non-specific binding of the probe, resulting in a high background noise and a reduced signal-to-noise ratio.

The sensitivity of ISH depends on the following variables: (a) the effect of tissue preparation on the retention and accessibility of target DNA or RNA; (b) the type of probe construction, including the efficiency of probe labelling and the sensitivity of the method used for signal detection; and (c) the effect of hybridization conditions on the efficiency of hybridization.

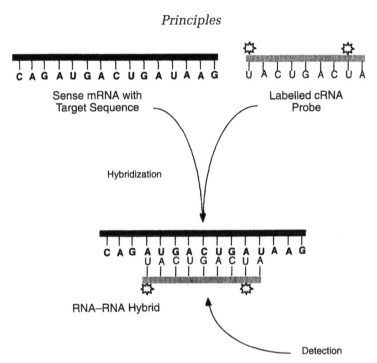

Fig. 1.1. Antisense RNA probe with labelled UTP hybridizing to a target sequence of mRNA (✿ represents the probe label).

Fixation and preparation of tissue

An optimal fixative for ISH must preserve a maximum level of target DNA or RNA while at the same time maintaining morphological detail and allowing access of the probe to its target. In contrast to the rather stable DNA, mRNA is normally steadily synthesized and enzymatically degraded within the cell. As a consequence, tissue to be used for RNA localization should be fixed or frozen as soon as possible after surgical excision, and the time between excision and adequate fixation has to be taken into account in each case when the results of ISH are interpreted (see section on interpretation of results). Whereas for DNA localization, the type and concentration of fixative is not of major importance, for RNA the localization, type, time, and concentration of the fixative are critical factors to avoid loss of RNA under the rigorous hybridization conditions of ISH. Paraformaldehyde, a cross-linking fixative, has been successfully used in many studies (Höfler *et al.* 1986; Jacobsson *et al.* 1996). Unlike other fixatives (e.g. glutaraldehyde), paraformaldehyde does not cross-link proteins as extensively and so allows penetration of even relatively long probes. Precipitating fixatives such as acetic acid–alcohol mixtures, or Bouin's fixation, have also been used for ISH (Evensen and Olesen 1997).

For mRNA localization we routinely fix tissue in buffered 4% paraformaldehyde for 1–2 h, followed by immersion in sucrose prior to freezing, to prevent freezing artefacts. The tissue is then kept in liquid nitrogen until cutting with a cryostat shortly before use. Alternatively, tissue can be snap frozen immediately after excision and stored, unfixed, in liquid nitrogen. Upon cryostat sectioning, tissue sections are briefly (10 min) fixed in 4% para-formaldehyde, air dried, and stores at −70 °C prior to hybridization. Although morphology with this latter method is not optimal, it has the advantage that the tissue can be used either for ISH or for extraction of DNA or RNA. Tissue sections and single cell preparations must be adhered to specially treated glass slides to avoid loss of tissue during the hybridization procedure. Gelatin–chromic alum coating of glass slides (Gall and Pardue 1971), treatment with poly-L-lysine (Huang *et al.* 1983), and, more recently, treatment with aminoalkylsilane (Rentrop *et al.* 1986) are some of the methods available for slide preparation.

Tissue fixation in formalin followed by paraffin embedding is the routine procedure in almost all pathology laboratories. DNA and mRNA with a high copy number can be detected in such tissues in most instances. The general reduction of hybridization efficiency in paraffin sections that has been observed may be a result of reduced accessibility of the probe to target DNA or RNA because of increased cross-linking of protein in paraffin sections compared with frozen sections (Campell and Habener 1987) or from loss of mRNA during the embedding procedure.

Pre-treatment of sections with a detergent and/or proteinase digestion is a standard procedure in almost all published ISH protocols and serves to increase probe penetration and accessibility, particularly with paraffin sections. Triton X-100 and RNAse-free proteinase K are commonly used, but pronase and pepsin are used in some protocols. A description of protocols for fixation and pre-treatment of cells for gene localization on chromosomes is beyond the scope of this chapter. For details and further references see Komminoth *et al.* (1994), Abati *et al.* (1995), and Cajulis *et al.* (1997), and Chapter 7.

Probes

Basically, labelled DNA and RNA probes can both be employed to localize DNA and mRNA (Table 1.1). There is general agreement that the optimal

Table 1.1 Probes for *in situ* hybridization

DNA	RNA
dsDNA	ss antisense RNA (cRNA)
vector or PCR derived	Synthetic oligonucleotides
Synthetic oligonucleotides	single or multiple
single or multiple	
ssDNA	

length of probes to allow for excellent tissue penetration and high hybridization efficiency is within the range 50–300 base pairs. For special applications such as localization of genes on chromosomes or when 'networking' for signal enhancement (Lawrence and Singer 1985), probes longer than 1.5 kb can be used, while probes shorter than 50 bp (oligonucleotides) are useful when closely related gene sequences must be distinguished from one another (Long *et al.* 1992).

Traditionally, the most frequently used probes were *double-stranded DNA (dsDNA)* (Fig. 1.2) probes, which are usually labelled by nick translation or random priming. *Nick translation* employs the enzymes DNase I and DNA polymerase I and can be performed with the specific insert only, or both the specific (insert) DNA and the plasmid vector. *Random priming* uses DNA with random primers, or calf thymus DNA with Klenow polymerase. Unlike nick translation, the double-stranded DNA template must be cut prior to labelling. Random priming allows the generation of probes with high specific activity but the yield of labelled probe is limited to approximately 50 ng for each synthesis reaction. Therefore, random priming reactions are not recommended for ISH studies in which large numbers of tissue sections are used, because approximately 10 ng of probe are required for each slide.

Synthetic oligodeoxyribonucleotides can be prepared conveniently by DNA synthesizers or by the PCR reaction and have several advantages over cloned DNA probes, including: (1) a consistently higher specific activity; (2) the

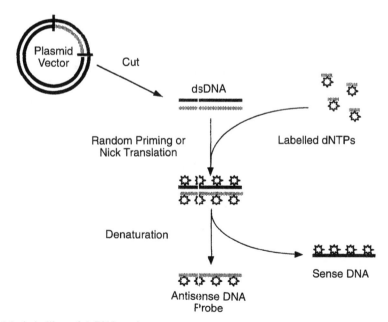

Fig. 1.2. Labelling of dsDNA probes.

possibility of synthesizing probes from amino acid sequences even when the total DNA sequence is unknown; (3) the ability to distinguish between closely homologous nucleic acid sequences; and (4) the opportunity to prepare several different probes directed at the same gene, a helpful control for hybridization specificity. Labelling of oligonucleotides is usually performed by *end-labelling techniques* either by 5′-end labelling with T4 polynucleotide kinase, or 3′-end labelling with terminal deoxynucleotidyl transferase (TdT). Oligonucleotides labelled with biotin (Larsson and Hougard, 1993) and digoxigenin (Crabb *et al.* 1992) have shown good results in several studies. The main disadvantage of oligonucleotide probes is their rather low specific activity. One method that has shown success in alleviating this problem is the use of mixtures of oligonucleotides directed at different sequences along the same gene (Fig. 1.3) (Harper *et al.* 1997).

With the introduction of the cloning vector M13 the generation of *single-stranded cDNA probes* (ssDNA) (Fig. 1.4) became possible (Varndell *et al.* 1984). The main reason for the restricted practical use of M13-derived ssDNA probes is probably the rather difficult vector construction and probe synthesis. More recently, this has been solved somewhat by the use of PCR-generated ssDNA probes of high specific activity (Katsahambas and Hearn 1996). Compared with double-stranded DNA, which has to be denatured prior to hybridization, these single-stranded probes have the advantage that reannealing of the probe to the second strand cannot occur (Schürch and Risau, 1991) and

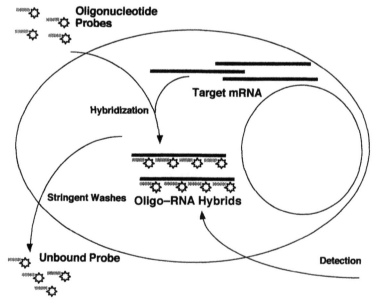

Fig. 1.3. Multiple oligonucleotide probes directed to different sequences along a segment of target mRNA.

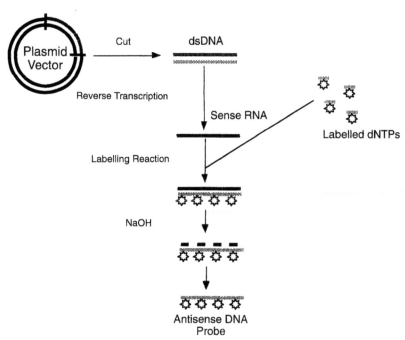

Fig. 1.4. Labelling of ssDNA probes.

they are not as 'sticky' as antisense RNA probes, thus yielding a sufficiently high signal-to-noise ratio for the demonstration of low copy number mRNA.

Cox *et al.* (1984) described a new approach employing *single-stranded antisense RNA probes* (ssRNA) generated from specially constructed RNA expression vectors, in a modification of a method originally introduced by Green *et al.* (1983). The advantages of antisense RNA probes over nick translated DNA probes include: (1) a higher specific activity; (2) the greater thermal stability of RNA–RNA hybrids; (3) a constant defined probe size; and (4) a lack of vector sequences within the probe that could lead to non-specific hybridization, all of which favour increased sensitivity and consistency of reactions. Furthermore, competitive hybridization to the complementary strand, as occurs with double-stranded probes, is excluded. Finally, and probably most importantly, is the ability to use RNase to digest non-hybridized (single-stranded) probe which provides an extremely low background. All the above-mentioned advantages result in extremely high sensitivity and excellent signal-to-noise ratios for ISH using cRNA probes. In addition, PCR can be modified to include a promoter sequence such as T7 in the segment to be amplified so that the resulting amplification product can be used as a template for the generation of ssRNA probes (Birk and Grimm 1994). Finally, through the use of subcloned synthetic oligonucleotides (20–70-mers) in RNA expression vectors, the synthesis of '*antisense RNA oligonucleotides*' is possible, thus combining the advantages of both oligonucleotide and cRNA probes.

Labelling

Two general strategies of probe labelling can be used: direct labelling, with direct attachment of the reporter molecule to DNA or RNA; and indirect labelling, in which either a hapten (e.g. biotin) is attached to the probe and detected by a labelled binding protein (e.g. avidin) or the probe–target hybrid is detected by a specific antibody. Currently available labelling methods for probes are summarized in Table 1.2.

Radioactively labelled probes, as originally developed by Gall and Pardue (1969), are still widely used for ISH, for several reasons, including: (1) the efficiency of probe synthesis can be more easily monitored; (2) radioisotopes are readily incorporated into synthesized DNA and RNA; and (3) high sensitivity, since autoradiography still represents the most sensitive detection system available. Signal detection can be achieved with autoradiography employing liquid emulsions or (with ^{32}P-labelled probes) X-ray films. Hydrogen-3 (^{3}H) is often used as a label because of the high resolution of the autoradiographs. Sections hybridized with ^{3}H-labelled probes, however, require a long exposure (weeks) for signal detection. If a more rapid detection is desired, labelling with high energy emitting radioisotopes, such as ^{32}P or ^{35}S, or, more recently, ^{33}P (Brimijoin and Hammond 1996) can yield auto-radiographs within days. Carbon-14 (^{14}C)- and ^{125}I-labelled probes are seldom used for ISH.

Problems of safety, waste disposal, and reduced stability of radioactively labelled probes, and speed of visualization, have directed attention to the

Table 1.2 Labelling of probes for *in situ* hybridization

Probe type	Label
Isotopic	^{3}H, ^{32}P, ^{33}P, ^{35}S, ^{14}C, ^{125}I
Non-isoptic	Alkaline phosphatase Biotin, photobiotin 5-Bromodeoxyuridine Dinitrophenyl (DNP) Ethidium Fluororescein Luciferase Mercury(II) acetate *N*-2-Acetylaminofluorene *N*-2-Acetylamino-7-iodofluorene Sodium metabisulfite Tetramethylrhodamine Antibodies directed to dsDNA, RNA–DNA, or RNA–RNAhybrids

development of *non-isotopic probes*. Among the choices for non-radioactive labels, biotin is currently favoured by many investigators since the detection system for biotin is well established in most laboratories on the basis of its widespread use in immunohistochemistry. With the synthesis of biotin-labelled dUTP (Langer *et al*. 1981), the construction of (directly) biotinylated nucleic acids (double-stranded DNA, single-stranded DNA, oligonucleotides, and cRNA) became possible. A problem with biotinylated probes is that, often, endogenous biotin cannot be blocked sufficiently and this results in high background noise. Other commonly used non-radioactive labels include alkaline phosphatase, digoxigenin, and 5-bromodeoxyuridine. Digoxigenin has shown good results and has good sensitivity, as well as good incorporation into either DNA or cRNA (Schaeren-Wiemers and Gerfin-Moser 1993), or oligonucleotide probes (Komminoth *et al*. 1992). Bromodeoxyuridine-labelled probes (Niedobitek *et al*. 1988) have good incorporation of label, but have disadvantages including low sensitivity because of reduced affinity of the antibody, and relative instability of the labelled probe. Particularly for viral detection by ISH, non-isotopic labelling using either biotin or digoxigenin is the method of choice.

Fluorescent labels for ISH (FISH) using fluorochrome-labelled DNA or RNA (Bauman 1985) are predominantly used for chromosomal ISH but are not otherwise widely used because of their relatively low sensitivity. However, some promising results have been obtained with chemiluminescence (Lorimer *et al*. 1993) which appears to have a level of sensitivity that may even exceed that of the other commonly used non-radioactive labels.

Sulfonated DNA probes for ISH were first described by Morimoto *et al*. (1987) and have the advantage of easy labelling. However, sulfonation can only be used for DNA probes, they have relatively high background and involve a long, complicated colour detection step.

Other probe labels based on chemically modified nucleic acids include, acetylaminofluorene (Landegent *et al*. 1984; Tchen *et al*. 1984), dinitrophenyl (DNP) groups as a hapten (Shroyer and Nakane 1983), mercurated probes and sulfhydryl–hapten ligands (Hopman *et al*. 1986) followed by immuno-histochemical detection with a labelled antibody. Direct detection of DNA–RNA or RNA–RNA hybrids by specific antibodies has also been employed by several groups in the past (Rudkin and Stollar 1977; Raap *et al*. 1984).

A rather new technique is oligonucleotide-primed *in situ* labelling (PRINS) which has been introduced for the detection of repetitive DNA sequences present in chromosomal centromeres or telomeres (Koch *et al*. 1989). PRINS is based on the hybridization of small oligonucleotides to repeated target sequences. The bound oligonucleotides provide multiple sites for the in-corporation of haptenized or directly fluorochrome-labelled nucleotides mediated by Taq polymerase. It has been shown that, in comparison to FISH, PRINS is faster and more cost effective (Koch *et al*. 1991; Gosden and Lawson 1994; Werner *et al*. 1997a). Whereas FISH can be applied to various tissue and cell preparations for the detection of chromosomal aberrations, PRINS has been mainly used for the analysis of chromosomal preparations that include nuclei of lysed cells. Recently, we were able to show that PRINS can also allow the demonstration of numerical karyotype changes in intact interphase cells prepared from various tissues (Wilkens *et al.* 1997; Werner *et al.* 1997a, b).

Modifications of the original PRINS reaction include multicolour PRINS, cycling PRINS, and 'instant' or 'flash' PRINS. The so-called multicolour PRINS (Volpi and Baldini 1993; Hindkjaer *et al.* 1994) allows for detection of more than one target sequence by repetition of the PRINS reaction. Different target sequences can be recognized by using differently labelled nucleotides. In cycling PRINS, the sensitivity of the reaction can be increased by performing multiple cycles of the reaction in the same reaction mixture. This method is useful when low copy number sequences are targeted (Gosden and Hanratty, 1993). Through the incorporation of directly flourochromatized nucleotides in the newly synthesized DNA, the time required for completion of a PRINS reaction can be reduced to 20 min (Gosden and Lawson 1994). This technique is referred to as 'instant' or 'flash' PRINS and can also be applied sequentially to label different targets (Speel *et al.* 1995). Another modification involves the enzymatic detection of incorporated nucleotides (Speel *et al.* 1995, 1997), with which chromosomes and cell morphology can be assessed with bright-field morphology.

Conditions of hybridization

One of the important advantages of ISH over immunohistochemistry is the fact that the degree of specificity of hybridization reactions can be accurately controlled by varying the reaction conditions. The degree of specificity depends on the construction of the probe, temperature, pH, the concentration of a denaturant such as formamide, and the concentration of salt in the hybridization buffer. One must be aware that, despite numerous mismatched bases along paired strands of nucleic acids, stable duplexes can form under certain hybridization conditions. The degree of mismatch that can be tolerated in hybridization reaction is referred to as its 'stringency'. Under conditions of high stringency, only probes with a high degree of homology to the target sequence will form stable hybrids. Under conditions of low stringency (i.e. reactions carried out at low temperature, in high salt, or at low formamide concentrations), a given probe may bind to sequences with only 70–90% homology, thus allowing for non-specific hybridization signals. Detailed studies concerning the influences of buffers, probe concentration, time, and temperature on hybridization efficiency for DNA probes (Lawrence and Singer 1985) and RNA probes (Höfler *et al.* 1986; Dirks *et al.* 1993) have been available for some time.

For ISH with radioactively labelled dsDNA or cRNA probes, 2–10 ng of probe diluted in hybridization buffer are usually applied per section. The volume of hybridization mixture should be kept as small as possible (i.e. 10–20 µl total volume per section covered with a 22 mm^2 coverslip). When biotinylated probes are used, 10–50 ng DNA probe per section are required. Most hybridization buffers contain a mixture of 50% formamide, 2 × SSC (standard saline citrate 1 × SSC = 0.15 M sodium chloride, 0.015 M sodium citrate). Dextran sulfate (usually 10%) can be added to increase hybridization efficiency (Wahl *et al.* 1979). Depending on the desired stringency and melting temperature of the hybrids, hybridization is carried out between 26 and 60 °C.

One of the major drawbacks of the ISH procedure, compared with hybridization reactions performed on extracts, is the limitation of hybridization and washing temperatures (and therefore stringency!) to temperatures no higher than 50 °C because of tissue damage and loss of sections from the slides at higher temperatures. Optimal annealing temperatures for cDNA and cRNA probes *in situ* are around 50 °C, i.e. 20–25 °C below their melting temperature (Cox *et al.* 1984). Hybridization reactions employing DNA probes may be completed after 4 h (Lawrence and Singer 1985), while reactions with cRNA probes should be incubated overnight. In contrast to the localization of mRNA, hybridization to cellular DNA requires the heating of tissue sections for 5–10 min at 90 °C to denature the target DNA. Washing steps to reduce non-specific binding are performed in decreasing concentrations of SSC (i.e. increasing stringency!), usually ending with 0.1 × SSC as the final wash step. For ISH employing radiolabelled probes, washing has to be rather extensive (up to several hours), whereas sections hybridized to non-radioactive probes require only a short washing procedure. RNase treatment of sections after hybridization with antisense RNA probes to decrease background appears to be more reliable than the comparable S1 nuclease treatment of DNA (Godard 1983). Prior to autoradiography with liquid emulsions, the sections must be air dried.

Interpretation of results

Specificity and sensitivity

As mentioned above, low stringency conditions may result in non-specific signals with ISH. Non-specific cross-hybridization occurs more often with long probes (> 0.5 kb) and with cRNA probes because of their higher affinity to DNA and RNA. Even under stringent reaction conditions, cross-hybridization of probes to related, but not identical, nucleic acid sequences containing highly homologous regions (e.g. gene families, such as HPC subtypes 6b and 11) is to be expected. Furthermore, non-specific binding to non-related genes and their messages as a result of partial sequence homology may occur (Crabbe 1985). One of the non-specific reactions that is most often seen in ISH for mRNA localization is the binding of probe to ribosomal RNA, which represents more than 90% of total cellular RNA. Because of the possibility of non-specific reactions, evaluation of each probe under different conditions of stringency is strongly recommended and, whenever possible, each probe should be tested by Northern blot analysis before it is used for ISH. Northern blots allow one to identify 'sticky' probes for which ISH results require a very cautious interpretation. Mast cells and eosinophils are another cause of non-specific ISH signals, probably because of ionic attraction of the probe to strongly charged compounds in the granules of these cells.

Besides non-specific binding of the probe, the detection system may also cause non-specific results. For example, the widely used biotinylated probes are usually immunohistochemically detected by avidin binding or by the application of biotin antibodies. In several tissues not probe bound but endogenous biotin may cause a strong 'non-specific' signal. Binding of biotin antibodies or avidin to endogenous biotin after ISH procedures cannot be prevented and represents a major restriction of the application of biotinylated probes. Chemography, the occurrence of spurious (non-radioactivity-induced) reaction products in the liquid emulsions used for the detection of radio-labelled probes, is caused by the interaction of heavy metal ions with the emulsion. Minimization or prevention of chemography can be achieved by: (1) omission of heavy metals from the fixatives; (2) exposure of slides at 4 °C; and (3) observance of constant temperature (15 °C) for Kodak NTB2, 20 °C for Ilford K2) during processing procedures. In systems using silver intensification, cross-reactions to the walls of fungi or pneumocystis organisms has been observed.

High sensitivity is one of the advantages of hybridization procedures, and can be exactly measured in all techniques in which tissue or cell extracts are used (e.g. blot hybridization). Similarly, the sensitivity of ISH in individual cells of homogeneous samples, such as cells grown in tissue culture, can be calculated based on the results of hybridization reactions on cell extracts. Using highly sensitive radiolabelled cRNA probes for mRNA detection, a sensitivity of 20 copies of mRNA per cell has been reported, which is approximately 10-fold higher than for ISH employing nick translated probes (Cox *et al.* 1984; Höfler *et al.* 1987a). These results were achieved in experiments under optimized conditions of fixation and hybridization and cannot be transferred to all experiments. The sensitivity of ISH, particularly for mRNA detection, on heterogeneous samples (i.e. tissue sections) cannot be monitored exactly. When the results of ISH are evaluated, the differing stability of individual species of mRNA must be considered. Delay in adequate tissue fixation after removal may lead to non-reproducible or even false negative results owing to mRNA degradation. Additionally, differences of accessibility of probes have been encountered in tissues from different organs. Interestingly, these differences appear to be restricted to oligonucleotide rather than cRNA probes (Campbell and Habener 1987).

Because of the relative stability of dsDNA, problems of loss, degradation, and reduced accessibility of the target sequences are usually not encountered when ISH is used to localize DNA. Furthermore, DNA target sequences on chromosomes are usually much longer and allow the use of longer (> 2 kb) probes. The sensitivity of ISH for DNA localization is therefore much higher than for RNA localization. Single copy genes can be detected in chromosomal preparations and, under certain circumstances, even in tissue sections.

Controls

As with all other histochemical methods, not every positive ISH signal is specific, and all available controls must be performed in order to prove specificity. Depending on the probe used and the target nucleic acid, several control methods are available (Table 1.3). Hybridization of the probe to extracted RNA or digested DNA after gel electrophoresis, and transfer on to solid supports (Northern or Southern blot analysis), should show hybridization to specific molecules of RNA or DNA only. These methods, which comparable to Western blot analysis for the control of antibody specificity, are the most important controls to assure probe specificity. Extracted DNA or RNA can also be used in slot blot hybridization as a control of probe sensitivity. When available, positive and negative cell lines or tissues provide evidence that the ISH reaction has the expected pattern of reactivity. If a suitable antibody is available, ISH and immunohistochemistry performed on serial or same sections (Höfler *et al.* 1987b; Denjin *et al.* 1992) can confirm that the mRNA is localized in cells containing the peptide product of the same gene. When immunohistochemistry cannot be done, hybridization with probes containing different specific sequences may be necessary. Similarly to pre-absorption of antibodies with specific antigens, pre-hybridization of probes with specific cDNA or cRNA should yield negative results of ISH. Furthermore, hybridization with non-specific vector sequences or sense RNA probes, should produce negative results. Alternatively, several probes directed to different sequences of the same gene can provide evidence of the specificity of the reaction. Another type of control is the use of non-complementary probes with the same length, which should yield a negative signal in comparison to

Table 1.3 Labelling of probes for *in situ* hybridization

Cell lines (positive and negative controls

Northern or Southern blots

Combination of ISH and immunohistochemistry

Hybridization with different probes complementary to the same target DNA or RNA

Blot hybridization to test probe sensitivity

Pre-hybridization of probe with cDNA or cRNA ('absorption')

Hybridization with non-homologous probes with similar length and GC content

Pre-treatment of sections with RNase or DNase

Emulsion or non-isotopic detection system controls

the specific probe. An example of such a control is the use of sense RNA probes generated from RNA expression vectors. Other controls include pre-treatment of sections with RNase or DNase to prove that the hybridization depends on the presence of RNA or DNA in the tissue. Finally, non-specific reactions in the detection system, such as chemography artefacts during autoradiography or non-specific reactions of the non-isotopic detection procedure, should be excluded by omitting the labelled probe in the protocol.

Conclusions and future aims

ISH represents a powerful method to localise DNA or RNA specifically in cells and is therefore able to provide valuable insights into differences in the biosynthetic activity of individual cells. Before commencing an experiment one must choose the appropriate system for probe construction, labelling, and signal detection. For the localization of DNA and high copy number mRNA, dsDNA probes or oligonucleotides, either radiolabelled or non-isotopically labelled are suitable. Isotopic labelling still represents the method of choice for the generation of probes, particularly cRNA probes, for the detection of low copy number mRNA by ISH, but non-isotopic methods are becoming increasingly more sensitive.

ISH can now be considered to be a routine technique for use in larger pathology laboratories. Its sensitivity, however, is limited, particularly in formalin-fixed material using non-isotopic methods for the detection of low copy number nucleic acids. In these cases the amplification of the target nucleic acid within the cell, either through the polymerase chain reaction (PCR) (Hasse *et al.* 1990; Komminoth *et al.* 1992; Nuovo *et al.* 1992), or, more recently, through self-sustained sequence replication (3SR) (Guatelli *et al.* 1990; Fahy *et al.* 1991; Hofler *et al.* 1995) can be applied. Alternatively, new methods are being developed that strongly increase the signal through amplification of the detection system. Examples of such methods include catalysed reporter depositions (CARD) with tyramide intensification of biotin signals (de Haas *et al.* 1996; Macechko, *et al.* 1997). Together, these developments hold the promise that, in the future, it will be possible to detect very low or even single copy numbers of mRNA or DNA in cells that until now have been below the detection limit of ISH.

Additional areas of progress in the future development of ISH include auto-mated systems for ISH, both for the technical execution of the reaction and the (semi-) automated histological evaluation of ISH results in cells or on slides.

References

Abati, A., Sandord, J.S., Fetsch, P., Marincola, F.M., and Wolman, S.R. (1995). Fluor-escence *in situ* hybridization (FISH): a user's guide to optimal preparation of cytologic specimens. *Diagn. Cytopathol.* **13**, 486–92.

Principles

Bauman, J.G.J. (1985). Fluorescence microscopical hybridocytochemistry. *Acta Histochem.* **31**, 9–18.

Biffo, S., Verdun-diCantogno, L., and Fasolo, A. (1992). Double labeling with non-isotopic *in situ* hybridization and BrdU immunohistochemistry: calmodulin (CaM) in mRNA expression in post-mitotic neurons of the olfactory system. *J. Histochem. Cytochem.*, **40**, 535–540.

Birk, P.E. and Grimm, P.C. (1994). Rapid nonradioactive in situ hybridization for interleukin-2 mRNA with riboprobes generated using the polymerase chain reaction. *J. Immunol. Meth.*, **167**, 83–9.

Brimijoin, S. and Hammond, P. (1996). Transient expression of acetylcholinesterase messenger RNA and enzyme activity in developing rat thalamus studied by quantitative histochemistry and *in situ* hybridization. *Neuroscience*, **71**, 555–65.

Buongiorno-Nardelli, M. and Amaldi, F. (1969). Autoradiographic detection of molecular hybrids between rRNA and DNA in tissue sections. *Nature* **225**, 946–7.

Cajulis, R.S., Yu, G. H., Cokaslan, S.T., and Hidvegi, D.F. (1977). Modified interphase cytogenetics technique as an adjunct in the analysis of atypical cells in body fluids. *Diagn. Cytopathol.*, **16**, 331–5.

Campbell, D.J. and Habener, J.F. (1987). Cellular localization of angiotensin gene expression in brown adipose tissue and mesentery: quantification of mRNA abundance using *in situ* hybridization. *Endocrinology*, **121**, 1616–26.

Cox, K.H., DeLeon, D.V., Angerer, L.M., and Angerer, R.C. (1984). Detection of mRNAs in sea urchin embryos by *in situ* hybridization using asymmetric RNA probes. *Dev. Biol.*, **101**, 485–502.

Crabb, I.D., Hughes, S.S., Hicks, D.G., Puzas, J.E., Tsao, G.J.Y., and Rosier, R.N. (1992). Nonradioactive *in situ* hybridization using dioxygenin-labeled oligodeoxynucleotides. *Am. J. Pathol.*, **141/3**, 579–89.

Crabbe, M.I. (1985). Partial sequence homologies between cytosceletal proteins, c-myc, Rous sarcoma virus and adenovirus proteins, transducin and beta- and gamma-crystalline. *Biosci. Rep.*, **5/2**, 167–74.

de Haas, R., Verwoerd, N.P., van der Corput, M., van Gijlswijk, R., Siitari, H., and Tanke, H.J. (1996). The use of peroxidase-mediated deposition of biotin-tyramide in combination with time-resolved fluorescence imaging of europium chelate label in immunohistochemistry and *in situ* hybridization. *J. Histochem. Cytochem.*, **44**, 1091–9.

Denjin, M., De Weger, R.A., Van Mansfeld, A.D.M., van Unnik, J.A.M., and Lips, C.J.M. (1992). Islet amyloid polypeptide (IAPP) is synthesized in the islets of langerhans. *Histochemistry*, **97**, 33–7.

Dirks, R.W., van de Rijke, F.M., Fujishita, S., van der Ploeg, M., and Raap, A.K. (1993). Methodologies for specific intron and exon RNA localization in cultured cells by haptenized and fluorochromized probes. *J. Cell. Sci.*, 1187–97.

Evensen, O., and Olesen, N.J. (1997). Immunohistochemical detection of VHS virus in paraffin-embedded specimens of rainbow trout (*Oncorhynchus mykiss*): the influence of primary antibody, fixative, and antigen unmasking on method sensitivity. *Vet. Pathol.*, **34**, 253–61.

Fahy, E., Kwoh, D.Y., and Gingeras, T.R. (1991). Self-sustained sequence replication (3SR): an isothermal transcription-based amplification system alternative to PCR. *PCR Meth. Appl.*, **1**, 25–33.

Gall, G. and Pardue, M.L., (1969). Formation and detection of RNA–DNA hybrid molecules in cytological preparations. *Proc. Natl. Acad. Sci. USA*, **63**, 378–81.

Gall, G. and Pardue, M.L. (1971). Nucleic acid hybridization in cytological preparations. *Meth. Enzymol.*, **38**, 470–80.

Godard, C.M. (1983). Improved method for detection of cellular transcripts by *in situ* hybridization. *Histochemistry*, **77**, 123–31.

Gosden, J. and Hanratty, D. (1993). PCR *in situ*: a rapid alternative to *in situ* hybridization for mapping short, low copy number sequences without isotopes. *Biotechniques*, **15**, 78–80.

Gosden, J. and Lawson, D. (1994). Rapid chromosome identification by oligonucleotide-primed *in situ* DNA synthesis (PRINS). *Hum. Mol. Genet.*, **3**, 931–6.

Green, M.R., Maniatis, T., and Melton, D.A. (1983). Human betaglobin pre-mRNA synthesized *in vitro* is accurately spliced in *Xenopus* oocyte nuclei. *Cell*, **32**, 681–94.

Guatelli, J.C., Whitfield, K.M., Kwoh, D.Y., Barringer, K.J., Richman, D.D., and Gingeras, T.R. (1990). Isothermal *in vitro* amplification of nucleic acids by a multienzyme reaction modeled after retroviral replication. *Proc. Natl. Acad. Sci. USA*, **87**, 1874–8.

Haase, A.T., Retzel, E.F., and Staskus, K.A. (1990). Amplification and detection of lentiviral DNA inside cells. *Proc. Natl. Acad. Sci. USA*, **87**, 4971–5.

Harper, S.J., Bailey, E., McKeen, C.M., Stewart, A.S., Pringle, J.H., Feehally, J., and Brown, T. (1997). A comparative study of digoxigenin, 2,4-dinitrophenyl, and alkaline phosphatase as deoxyoligonucleotide labels in non-radioisotopic *in situ* hybridization. *J. Clin. Pathol.*, **50**, 686–90.

Hindkjaer, J., Koch, J., Terkelsen, C., Brandt, C.A., Kolvaa, S., and Bolund, L. (1994). Fast, sensitive multicolor detection of nucleic acids in situ by PRimed IN Situ labeling (PRINS). *Cytogenet. Cell. Genet.*, **66**, 152–4.

Höfler, H. (1987). *In situ* hybridization. A review. *Path. Res. Pract.*, **182**, 421–30.

Höfler, H., Childers, H., Montminy, M.R., Lechan, R.M., Goodman, R.H., and Wolfe, H.J. (1986). *In situ* hybridization methods for the detection of somatostatin mRNA in tissue sections using antisense RNA probes. *Histochem. J.*, **18**, 597–604.

Höfler, H., Childers, H., Montminy, M.R., Goodman, R.H., Lechan, R.M., DeLellis, R.A., Tischler, A.S., and Wolfe, H.J. (1987a). Localization of somatostatin mRNA in the gut, pancreas and thyroid gland of the rat using antisense RNA probes for *in situ* hybridization. *Acta. Histochem. Suppl.*, **XXXIV**, 101–5.

Höfler, H., Ruhri, Ch., Pütz, B., Wirnsberger, G., Klimpfinger, M., and Smolle, J. (1987b). Simultaneous localization of calcitonin mRNA and peptide in a medullary thyroid carcinoma. *Virch. Arch. B.*, **53/3**, 144–51.

Höfler, H., Putz, B., Mueller, J.D., Neubert, W., Sutter, G., and Gais, P. (1995). *In situ* amplification of measles virus RNA by the self-sustained sequence replication reaction. *Lab. Invest.* **73**, 577–85.

Hopman, A.H.N., Wiegant, J., and Duijn, P. van (1986). A new hybridocytochemical method based on mercurated nucleic acid probes and sulfhydril–hapten ligands. I. Stability of mercury–sulfhydril bond and influence of the ligand structure on immunochemical detection detection of the hapten. *Histochemistry*, **84**, 169–78.

Huang, W.M., Gibson, S.J., Facer, P., Gu, J., and Polak, J.M. (1983). Improved section adhesion for immunohistochemistry using high molecular weight polymers of L-lysine as a slide coating. *Histochemistry*, **77**, 275–9.

Jacobsson, B., Bernell, P., Arvidsson, I., and Hast, R. (1996). Classical morphology, esterase cytochemistry, and interphase cytogenetics of peripheral blood and bone marrow smears. *J. Histochem. Cytochem.*, **44**, 1303–9.

John, H.L., Birnstiel, M.L., and Jones, K.W. (1969). RNA–DNA hybrids at the cytological level. *Nature*, **223**, 912–13.

Katsahambas, S., and Hearn, M.T. (1996). Localization of basic fibroblast growth factor mRNA (FGF-2 mRNA) in the uterus of mated and unmated gilts. *J. Histochem. Cytochem.*, **44**, 1289–301.

Koch, J., Kolvraa, S., Petersen, K.B., Gregersen, N., and Bolund, L. (1989). Oligonucleotide-priming methods for the chromosome-specific labelling of alpha satellite DNA *in situ*. *Chromosoma*, **98**, 259–65.

Koch, J., Hindkjaer, J., Mogensen, J., Kolvraa, S., and Bolund, L. (1991). An improved method for chromosome-specific labeling of alpha satellite DNA *in situ* by using denatured double-stranded DNA probes as primers in a primed *in situ* labeling (PRINS) procedure. *Genet. Anal. Tech. Appl.*, **8**, 171–8.

Komminoth, P., Long, A.A., Ray, R., and Wolfe, H.J. (1992). *In situ* polymerase chain reaction detection of viral DNA, single copy genes and gene rearrangements in cell suspensions and cytospins. *Diagn. Mol. Pathol.*, **1**, 85–97.

Komminoth, P., Adams, V., Long, A.A., Roth, J., Saremaslani, P., Flury, R., Schmid, M., and Heitz, P.U., (1994). Evaluation of methods for hepatitis C virus detection in archival liver biopsies. Comparison of histology, immunohistochemistry, *in situ* hybridization, reverse transcriptase polymerase chain reaction (RT-PCR) and *in situ* RT-PCR. *Pathol. Res. Pract.*, **190**, 1017–25.

Landegent, J.E., Jansen, I.N., de Wal, N., Baan, R.A., Hoeymakers, J.H.J., and van der Pleog, M. (1984). 2-Acetylaminofluorene-modified probes for the indirect hybrido-chemical detection of specific nucleic acid sequences. *Exp. Cell. Res.*, **153**, 61–72.

Langer, P.R., Waldrop, A.A., and Ward, D.C. (1981). Enzymatic synthesis of biotin-labeled polynucleotides: novel nucleic acid affinity probes. *Proc. Natl. Acad. Sci. USA*, **78/11**, 6633–7.

Larsson, L.I. and Hougard, (1993). Sensitive detection of rat gastrin mRNA by *in situ* hybridization with chemically biotynlated oligodeoxynucleotides: validation, quanitiation and double staining studies. *J. Histochem. Cytochem.*, **41**, 157–163.

Lawrence, J.B. and Singer, R.H. ((1985). Quantitative analysis of *in situ* hybridiz-ation methods for the detection of actin gene expression. *Nucl. Acids Res.*, **13/5**, 1777–99.

Long, A.A., Mueller, J.D., Andre-Schwartz, Barrett, K.J., Schwartz, R., and Wolfe, H.J. (1992). High specificity *in situ* hybridization. *Diagn. Mol. Pathol.*, **1**, 45–57.

Lorimer, P., Lamarq, F., Labat-Moluer, C., Guillermet, C., Bethier, R., and Stoebner, P. (1993). Enhanced chemiluminescence: a high-sensitivity detection system for *in situ* hybridization and immunohistochemistry. *J. Histochem. Cytochem.*, **41**, 1591–7.

Macechko, P.T., Krueger, L., Hirsch, B., and Erlandsen, S.L. (1997). Comparison of immunologic amplification vs enzymatic deposition of fluorochrome-conjugated tyramide as detection systems for FISH. *J. Histochem. Cytochem.* **45**, 359–63.

Morimoto, H., Monden, T., Shimano, T., Higashiyama, M., Tomita, N., Murotani, M., Matsuura, N., Okuda, H., and Mori, T. (1987). Use of sulfonated probes in *in situ* detection of amylase mRNA in formalin-fixed paraffin sections of human pancreas and submaxillary gland. *Lab. Invest.*, **57/6**, 737–41.

Niedobitek, G., Finn, T., Herbst, H., Bornhöft, G., Gerdes, J., and Stein, H. (1988).

Detection of viral DNA by *in situ* hybridization using bromodeoxyuridine-labeled DNA probes. *Am. J. Pathol.*, **131/1**, 1–4.

Nuovo, G.J., Becker, J., Margiotta, M., MacConnell, P., Comite, S., and Hochman, H. (1992). Histological distribution of polymerase chain reaction-amplified human papillomavirus 6 and 11 in penile lesions. *Am. J. Surg. Pathol.*, **16**, 269–75.

Raap, A.K., Marijnen, J.G.J., and van der Ploeg, M. (1984). Anti-DNA.RNA sera. Specifity test and application in quantitative *in situ* hybridization. *Histochemistry*, **81**, 517–20.

Rentrop, M., Knapp, B., Winter, H., and Schweizer, J. (1986). Aminoalkysilane treated glass slides as support for *in situ* hybridization of keratin cDNAs to frozen tissue sections under varying fixation and pretreatment conditions. *Histochem. J.*, **18**, 271–6.

Rudkin, G.T. and Stollar, B.D. (1977). High resolution detection of DNA–RNA hybrids *in situ* by indirect fluorescence. *Nature*, **265**, 472–3.

Schaeren-Wiemers, N. and Gerfin-Moser, A. (1993). A single protocol to detect transcripts of various types and expression levels in neural tissue and cultured cells: *in situ* hybridization using digoxigenin-labelled cRNA probes. *Histochemistry*, **100**, 431–40.

Schürch, H. and Risau, W. (1991). Differentiating and mature neurons express the acidic fibroblast growth factor gene during chick neural development. *Development*, **111**, 1143–54.

Shroyer, K.P. and Nakane, P.K.J. (1983). Use of DNP-labeled cDNA for *in situ* hybridization. *J. Cell Biol.*, **97**, 377a.

Speel, E.J., Lawson, D., Hopman, A.H., and Gosden, J. (1995). Multi-PRINS: multiple sequential oligonucleotide primed *in situ* DNA synthesis reactions label specific chromosomes and produce hands. *Hum. Genet.*, **95**, 29–33.

Speel, E.J., Lawson, D., Ramaekers, F.C., Gosden, J.R., and Hopman, A.H. (1997). Bright-field microscopic detection of oligonucleotide PRINS-labeled DNA in chromosome preparations. *Meth. Mol. Biol.*, **71**, 13–22.

Tchen, P., Fuchs, R.P.P., Sage, E., and Leng, M. (1984). Chemically modified nucleic acids as immunodetectable probes in hybridization experiments. *Proc. Natl. Acad. Sci. USA*, **81**, 3466–70.

Varndell, I.M., Polak, J.M., Sikri, K.L., Minth, C.D., Bloom, S.R., and Dixon, J.E. (1984). Visualisation of messenger RNA directing peptide synthesis by *in situ* hybridization using a novel single-stranded cDNA probe. *Histochemistry*, **81**, 597–601.

Volpi, E. and Baldini, A. (1993). MULITPRINS: a method formulticolor primed *in situ* labeling. *Chrom. Res.*, **1**, 257–60.

Wahl, G.M., Stern, M., and Stark, G.R. (1979). Efficient transfer of large fragments from agarose gels to diazobenzyloxymethyl-paper and rapid hybridization by using dextran sulfate. *Proc. Natl. Acad. Sci. USA*, **76**, 3683–7.

Werner, M., Wilkens, L., Nasarek, A., Tchinda, J., and Komminoth, P. (1997a). Detection of karyotype changes in interphase cells: oligonucleotide- primed *in situ* labelling versus fluorescence *in situ* hybridization. *Virch. Arch.*, **430**, 381–7.

Werner, M., Ewig, M., Nasarek, A., Wilkens, L., von Wasielewski, R., Tchinda, J., and Nolte, M. (1997b). Value of fluorescence *in situ* hybridization (FISH) for detecting bcr/abl gene fusion in interphase cells of routine bone marrow specimens. *Diagn. Mol. Pathol.*, **430**, 381–7.

Wilkens, L., Komminoth, P., Nasarek, A., von W.R., and Werner, M. (1997). Rapid detection of karyotype changes in interphase bone marrow cells by oligonucleotide primed *in situ* hybridization (PRINS). *J. pathol.*, **181**, 368–73.

Wolfe, K.Q. and Herrington, C.S. (1997). Interphase cytogenetics and pathology: a tool for diagnosis and research. *J. Pathol.*, **181**, 359–61.

2

The design and generation of probes for *in situ* hybridization

MARY E. SUNDAY

Introduction and overview of probes

The design and generation of probes for *in situ* hybridization (ISH) are critical determinants for the successful outcome of every experiment. It is necessary to use a labelled hybridization probe to detect the mRNA of interest in the target tissue section. There is no concern that nuclear DNA might also hybridize, because the double-stranded DNA is not denatured and thus not available for hybridization in mRNA ISH protocols. A variety of probes can be used, and they can be synthesized in different ways. Most often, radio-labelled probes are used together with autoradiography, but new methods of detecting non-isotopic probes are becoming widely used (see section on probe labelling below).

To optimize an ISH protocol, high stringency conditions are generally used during hybridization of a probe, including low salt concentration and high concentration of formamide in the hybridization buffer and high temperature during the hybridization and washing steps (Ausubel *et al.* 1987; Davis *et al.* 1986). Consequently, nucleic acid probes yield the best results if the probe and tissue sections are from the same species. Although a highly homologous (over 90% identical base pairs) probe may work perfectly well, the outcome may, none the less, be negative. The first step in designing a probe for ISH may therefore be the cloning and sequencing of a partial or full-length cDNA homologous to the species of the tissues being investigated. This hurdle has been greatly simplified with the advent of polymerase chain reaction (PCR) technology (discussed below). Usually, with homologous probes, it does not matter whether coding or non-coding segments of cDNA are selected, provided that regions containing repetitive sequences are avoided. In designing a cross-species probe. it is a good rule of thumb to select coding regions that include highly conserved sequences, if this information is available, because 5'-UT and 3'-UT regions may be less conserved than the coding regions (Eldridge *et al.* 1985).

Nucleic acid probes are of three general types: cRNA, cDNA, and oligo-

Table 2.1 Nucleic acid probes

Probe type	Advantages	Disadvantages
cRNA	Both antisense and sense probes available, providing internal negative control	Both antisense and sense strands may be transcribed (Miyajuma *et al.* 1989)
	Uniform length	Need to obtain cDNA and/or
	High affinity of RNA–RNA hybrids	subclone into appropriate
	Low background with RNase as a	plasmid vector
	post-hybridization treatment	Labile
cDNA	Stable	High background
	Probe 'networking' amplifies signal	Need to obtain cDNA
Oligonucleotide	Ready source, requires only sequence data	Lower signal-to-noise ratio
	Sense and scrambled controls available	

nucleotide probes (Table 2.1). Each of these will be discussed in detail (see later). In the literature, cRNA and oligonucleotide probes are most widely used for detecting low abundance and high abundance mRNAs, respectively. All three types of nucleic acid probe can be labelled using isotopic or non-isotopic methods. The details of our entire ISH protocol have been published previously (Spindel *et al.* 1987; Sunday *et al.* 1988, 1991; Sunday 1991).

Probe labelling: radioactive versus non-radioactive

The choice of labelling method depends first on whether the target mRNA is of high abundance or low abundance in the tissue being investigated. Radioactive labelling remains the method of choice for most laboratories for low abundance mRNAs, because it is the most sensitive indicator when conditions are optimized, yielding about a three to four times higher signal-to-noise ratio in our experience (Höfler *et al.* 1988; Sunday 1991). High abundance mRNAs such as those encoding actin or high abundance growth factors, may be detected using either radioactive or non-radioactive probes (Singer and Ward 1982; Humpel *et al.* 1993). Because ISH is mainly a technique for scientific inquiry rather than a clinical laboratory procedure, the use of isotopic labelling remains widespread. The major agents that have been utilized in probe labelling are summarized in Table 2.2.

With regard to isotopic probes, ^{35}S has been the most widely used, for several reasons.

1. The beta rays emitted by ^{3}H and ^{35}S are of lower average energy (average beta 0.0057 and 0.0488 MeV, respectively) than those from ^{32}P (0.695 MeV

Table 2.2 Agents for probe labelling

	Half-life	Scatter	Time to results	Hazard
^{32}P	14.3 days	High	Days to weeks	Moderate
^{33}P	25.4 days	Lower	Days to weeks	Moderate
^{35}S	87.4 days	Low	Weeks	Low
^{3}H	12 years	None	Weeks to months	Very low
Biotin	N/A	None	1–3 days	None*
Digoxigenin	N/A	None	1–3 days	None*

*The non-isotopic methods pose a health hazard when carcinogenic substrates are used for developing, such as diaminobenzidine for the immunoperoxidase method.

average) (Shapiro 1981), and so are less of a health hazard and yield better autoradiographic cell-specific localization.

2. Because of their longer half-life and lower energy emissions, which do not break the cRNA molecule into smaller fragments at the site of isotopic disintegration, ^{35}S-labelled probes may be stored at $-70°C$ indefinitely, as long as the cRNA has not been degraded. In contrast, ^{32}P-labelled probes must be used within 1–3 days of synthesis.

3. The exposure time required for an optimal signal-to-noise ratio is generally 7–9 days, which is comparable with that for ^{32}P, and much shorter than that for ^{3}H (Table 2.2).

Phosphorus-33 (^{33}P) is a newly developed isotope that has properties comparable with ^{35}S and which is technically superior to either ^{32}P or ^{35}S for ISH (Johnston *et al.* 1997), even though it is more expensive(Evans and Read 1992; Baskin and Stahl 1993; Biroc *et al.* 1993; Humpel *et al.* 1993; McLaughlin and Margolskee 1993; Jostarndt *et al.* 1994). The main advantage of ^{33}P over ^{35}S is that it results in 10-fold less non-specific background hybridization than ^{35}S, which can be important for detection of low abundance mRNAs (McLaughlin and Margolskee 1993).

Although ^{3}H-labelled probes yield the best cell-specific localization, compared with probes labelled with any of the other radioisotopes, the long time period required for exposure of autoradiograms makes this a less desirable agent.

Non-radiolabelled probes are more widely used than ^{3}H-labelled probes when exact, cell-specific localization is critical, because the time to obtaining results is no more than 3 days, compared with 3 weeks to 3 months or longer for ^{3}H (Niedobitek *et al.* 1989; Pang and Baum 1993; Yameda *et al.* 1994). Non-isotopic probes are being used increasingly, usually for high abundance mRNAs and also because of their superior safety and the speed of obtaining results. In the literature, there are also descriptions of the use of such probes for detecting low abundance mRNAs, such as the gastrin-releasing peptide receptor in human fetal lung (Wang and Cutz 1994). Labelling of cDNAs or cRNAs may be carried out by the incorporation of biotinylated-UTP or -dUTP (Singer and Ward 1982; Niedobitek *et al.* 1989; Dirks *et al.* 1991) or digoxigenin-11-UTP or -dUTP (Dirks *et al.* 1991; Komminoth 1992; Humpel *et al.* 1993; Pang and Baum 1993; Yamada *et al.* 1994) (and according to the manufacturer's specifications, Boehringer Mannheim Corp., Indianapolis, IN) in place of radiolabelled-UTP or -dCTP (Sunday 1991). As an alternative, cold cRNAs, cDNAs, or oligonucleotides can be biotinylated directly using photo-biotin (Vector Laboratories) according to the manufacturer's specifications (Forster *et al.* 1985; Khan and Wright 1987; Chantratita *et al.* 1989; McInnes *et al.* 1990).

A combination of biotinylated and digoxigenin-labelled probes, or of isotopic and non-isotopic probes, may be used for detecting multiple mRNAs in the same tissue section (Dirks *et al.* 1991; Wang and Cutz 1994). Similarly, ISH may be carried out in the same tissue section as a parallel immuno-histochemical reaction if the reaction products are different (Steel *et al.* 1988; van den Brunk *et al.* 1990). However, a strongly positive autoradiograph signal may be of such high grain density as to obscure the cytoplasm, so that a non-isotopic detection would be rendered uninterpretable. Similarly, it may be difficult to confirm double labelling of a given cell with double non-isotopic detection when the cell is strongly positive for two gene products. An accept-able alternative to double labelling in the same tissue section is to carry out ISH using thin serial sections in parallel with two different probes, or ISH and immunohistochemistry in parallel serial sections (Spindel *et al.* 1987; Sunday *et al.* 1988; Sunday 1991).

Experimental strategy and probe selection

The anticipated abundance of target mRNAs in tissue sections is often the major determinant of the type of probe to be used for ISH. Hence, cRNAs are the probe of choice for analyses of low abundance mRNAs, the kinetics of appearance of mRNAs during developmental processes, or pilot experiments analysing the cell-specific distribution of novel mRNAs (Spindel *et al. 1987; Sunday* et al. 1988; Sunday 1991; Black *et al.* 1993; Jostarndt *et al.* 1994). The use of cRNAs also offers other advantages (Table 2.1): the affinity of RNA–RNA hybrids is high and the background binding of single-stranded cRNAs to other chemical moieties is abolished during the post-hybridization washes by treatment with RNase A (Ausubel *et al.* 1987). The major dis-advantage of using cRNAs is their lability, which requires special precautions to avoid contamination with the ubiquitous RNases prior to or during hybrid-ization. Although one does need a cDNA subcloned into an appropriate vector containing an RNA polymerase promoter, this is a small obstacle if a cDNA is available or can be generated by PCR. The uniform length of cRNAs synthesized using a given plasmid template also favours low back-ground noise. cRNAs as small as 100 bp can be used, but our best results have been with probes 150–700 bp in length. cRNA probes greater than 700 bp do not penetrate tissue sections easily, but can be treated with alkaline hydrolysis to achieve an average fragment size of less than 250 bp prior to hybridization (Wada *et al.* 1993). cRNA probes have a further advantage of availability of the sense cRNA as a negative control (see below).

cDNA probes have been the method of choice for chromosomal DNA ISH protocols to localize genes, and can also be used for ISH when the mRNA of interest is known to be highly abundant (Khan and Wright 1987; Chantratita *et al.* 1989). For either DNA or RNA ISH protocols, the phenomenon of 'networking', whereby the sense and antisense strands bind to each other in a staggered fashion, leads to amplification of the signal (Table 2.1). These probes have the advantage of being chemically stable because contamination with DNases (which are heat labile) is less of a problem than that with RNases (which even survive boiling). However, many of the cDNAs synthesized during labelling with either nick translation or the random priming method are small fragments (less than 100 bp) which have a greater tendency to bind non-specifically and increase the background noise. Furthermore, the sense and antisense strands are both synthesized in the probe reaction, so the sense control is not available. cDNA prepared from vector alone is an alternative negative control. The need for a cDNA template is not a major concern since the advent of PCR cloning techniques, provided the sequence is available.

Oligonucleotides are readily available, bypassing the need for a cDNA, but do yield a lower signal-to-noise ratio because they are usually only 40 bp or less in size and are end-labelled and of lower specific activity than cRNA or random-primed cDNA probes (see below) (Ausubel *et al.* 1987; Long *et al.* 1992; Biroc *et al.* 1993). There may also be more non-specific binding of oligonucleotides to specific cell types, such as neuroendocrine cells (Pagani *et al.* 1993). Hence, they are usually only used to detect higher abundance mRNAs. Sense and scrambled negative controls are both available and would be useful to resolve whether the signal is real or represents non-specific binding.

For ISH to detect transgene expression, the probe of choice should be entirely transgene specific without any cross-hybridization to the corresponding or related endogenous genes. Therefore, a probe to detect the SV40 poly(A) tail in transgene-derived transcripts would be of general usefulness for any transgene using this sequence as a polyadenylation signal.

The specific activity of radiolabelled probes can be determined by a comparison of the radioactivity incorporated with the total input radioactivity in an aliquot of the reaction. For cRNA and random-primed cDNA probes, the specific activity is usually greater than 109 dpm/μg.

cRNA probe labelling

The cDNA fragment of interest should be subcloned preferentially into one of the pGEM or Bluescript vectors, which allows one to generate both

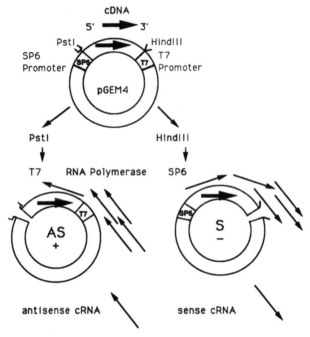

Fig. 2.1. cRNA probe labelling.

antisense and control sense probes from the same subclone, as indicated in Fig. 2.1. First, the cDNA template must be linearized at one end of the insert to limit the length of the probe to the insert size (or smaller, if desired and restriction sites permit). A typical restriction digest would be set up as follows (Ausubel *et al.* 1987).

(i)   100 μg of circular plasmid containing cDNA,

(ii)   in 85 μl of DEPC-treated autoclaved deionized H$_2$O,

(iii)   + 10 μl of the appropriate 10 × buffer

(iv)   + 5 μl of enzyme (10–20 units/μl)

After incubation for 2 h at 37 °C, enzyme is inactivated at 65 °C for 5 min to stop its exonuclease activity. Linearized cDNA is purified by ethanol precipitation (add 11 μl of 3.0 M sodium acetate and 222 μl of 100% ethanol, chilling on dry ice for 20 min, spinning in a microcentrifuge for 20 min at 4 °C, and resuspended in 50 μl of sterile H$_2$O).

The cRNA probe reaction is set up as follows.

(i)   250 μCi of 35S-UTP (New England Nuclear #NEG-039H, specific activity 1000–1500 Ci/mmol) is desiccated in a siliconized sterile microcentrifuge tube (1.5 μl capacity). To this is added, sequentially,

(ii)   1 μl of linearized template (1–2 μg)

(iii) 2 μl of 5 × RNA polymerase buffer (comes with the enzyme)

(iv)   2 μl of ATP+CTP+GTP containing 2.5 mM each

(v)   1 μl of dithiothreitol (DTT, 100 mM stock)

(vi)   1 μl of RNasin

(vii) 2 μl DEPC-treated H_2O

(viii) 1 μl of the appropriate RNA polymerase

(We have used Promega as the source of reagents for this reaction).

   After incubation at 37°C for 90 min, the cRNA probe is ready for ethanol precipitation, which can be achieved by adding, sequentially,

(i)   1 μl (10 μg/ml) of yeast tRNA as carrier

(ii)   1.3 μl of 3.0 M sodium acetate

(iii) 50 μl of 100% ethanol

   For calculations of specific activity, the amount of cRNA, in μg, generated during this reaction can be estimated by comparing an aliquot of the probe on an ethidium bromide-stained agarose gel with known standards of control DNA (5% of the probe prior to ethanol precipitation in one lane versus a control DNA insert of similar size at 10, 25, 50, 100, and 200 ng per lane).

   We have found it unnecessary to remove the cDNA template prior to precipitation, because it in no way interferes with the subsequent hybridization of the cRNA probe (Sunday 1991).

   If the cRNA is greater than 600–700 bp, alkaline hydrolysis can be carried out to reduce the average probe size to less than 250 bp to improve the penetration of tissue sections by probe (Wada *et al.* 1993). However, in our experience this leads to partial degradation of the probe and hence a weaker signal-to-noise ratio. Thus, our preferred protocol is to use a cRNA probe that is less than 600 bp.

   cRNAs must be stored at −70°C or less to avoid degradation.

Oligonucleotide probe labelling

The most widely used method of labelling oligonucleotides is end-labelling with T4 polynucleotide kinase (Ausubel *et al.* 1987; Davis *et al.* 1988). A typical reaction would be set up as follows.

(i)   Take 1.0 μl of oligonucleotide (0.5 μg)

(ii)   Add 2.5 μl of 10 × kinase buffer (500 mM Tris, pH 7.4; 100 mM $MgCl_2$; 50 mM DTT)

(iii) Add 20 μl gamma-^{35}S-ATP (3000 Ci/mmol; 10 μCi/μl)

(iv)   Add 1.5 μl T4 kinase

The reaction is allowed to incubate for 45 min at 37°C, then stopped for 5 min at 65°C. For ISH, the probe should be ethanol precipitated as described for CRNA probe labelling and then stored at either −20 or −70°C.

cDNA probe labelling

Nick translation, the original method for cDNA labelling has now been superceded by the random priming method, which reproducibly yields cDNA probes of high specific activity, most of which range from 500 to 600 bp (Ausubel *et al.* 1987). The protocols are usually supplied together with all the required reagents (excluding the cDNA template) in kits. We have used the Boehringer Mannheim kit most often and have found it to be almost foolproof. In brief, the protocol we use is as follows.

(i)   To 7 μl of sterile deionized H_2O containing 25 to 250 ng cDNA

(ii) Add 2 μl of random primers (50 ng/μl)

Pipette into a screw-cap siliconized microfuge tube. Denature the DNA by heating for 10 min at 95°C and subsequent cooling on ice. Add, sequentially,

(i)   3 μl dATP+dGTP+dTTP (0.5 mM each)

(ii)   2 μl DTT (20 mM stock)

(iii) 2 μl 10 × random primer buffer (900 mM HEPES pH 6.6/100 mM $MgCl_2$)

(iv)   5 μl [alpha-^{35}S]dCTP (10 μCi/μl. 3000 ci/mmol aqueous solution)

(v)   1 μl Klenow fragment of DNA polymerase 1 (~5 units) Incubate for 1 h at 37°C, or 16 h at room temperature (add a second 1 μl aliquot of Klenow after 5 h of incubation at room temperature to boost the specific activity even further). The reaction can be stopped by heating to 65°C for 10 min. Ethanol precipitate the probe as described above. The specific activity should be greater than 10^9 dpm/μg.

Probes from PCR-generated fragments

Prior to the advent of PCR technology, the rate-determining step in initiating an ISH project was the availability of or access to the cDNA of interest from the same species as the tissue being investigated. Even then, smaller cDNA fragments less than 700 bp were clearly more advantageous for generating cRNA probes to penetrate tissue sections, but the appropriate restriction endonuclease sites were not present. Denny *et al.* (1988) described an alternative route using synthetic oligodeoxynucleotides to generate short (<50 bp) single-stranded cRNA probes ('oligoriboprobes') which could be of further usefulness in identifying cells producing closely related but distinct mRNAs. However, although innovative, this approach is limited by the time required to generate the oligonucleotides and its limitation to species for which precise sequence information is available.

PCR technology has bypassed many of these obstacles (Eisenstein 1990; Erlich *et al.* 1991). Oligonucleotide primers can be designed to span almost any region of interest provided that some sequence information is available, for as little as 50 bp up to 2000–3000 bp. If the primers correspond to highly conserved segments of DNA, PCR can be carried out in diverse species, so that an homologous cDNA may be generated from the same species as the tissue being examined. Computerized programs are available for designing optimal PCR primers. PCR products may be subcloned either by including specific restriction enzyme sites at opposite ends of the insert, or using a commercially available kit (Invitrogen, Stratagene, Promega, and others). We have had the best results using Stratagene's kit for direct subcloning of PCR products. The vector that the PCR products are cloned into should contain at least one RNA polymerase promoter for subsequent generation of cRNA probes for ISH. To ensure that the probe indeed corresponds to the gene of interest, direct sequencing of the PCR products may be carried out. Alternatively, a Southern blot of the PCR products may be probed using an independent, third internal oligonucleotide with high stringency conditions.

PCR may also be utilized to identify new probes of interest that may be differentially expressed in a tissue-specific fashion or developmentally regulated. For a more detailed discussion of PCR protocols and applications, the reader is referred to recent reviews on this subject (Eisenstein 1990; Erlich *et al.* 1991).

Controls

Control probes for ISH are an important component of every experiment for ruling out the possibility of artefactual signals, such as at the edges of the tissue section, or overlying grains of talc. The ideal negative control probe is one of the same length(s), the same GC content, and labelled in parallel with the same agent. The controls most often used for the different types of probe are as follows.

(a) Antisense cRNA probes are complementary to mRNAs in the tissue sections and hence should hybridize. Their ideal negative control is the sense cRNA, which is identical to tissue mRNAs and hence should not hybridize. The only caveat here is that occasionally both sense and antisense strands of DNA are transcribed (Miyajima *et al.* 1989). If one observes a positive hybridization signal using negative control probes, it is advisable to probe identical Northern blots of control tissues in parallel to see whether any bands are observed (although a negative Northern blot would not conclusively rule out this possibility). As a back-up, one can, instead, use a cRNA prepared from the bacterial pGEM or Bluescript vector that clearly should not exist in mammalian tissues. In this case, the probe should be close to the same length and GC content as the antisense probe.

(b) For antisense oligonucleotide probes, the ideal control is a scrambled oligonucleotide of the same length and nucleotide content, but with 3 or 4 nucleotides shuffled around such that it represents a nonsense probe. An alternative would be the corresponding sense probe of the same length.

(c) For cDNA probes, which by definition are double-stranded, including both antisense and sense sequences, the major negative controls are other cDNAs that are known to be negative by RT-PCR in the tissue(s) of interest.

(d) For any probe type, a negative control probe would be one known to be absent from the tissue of interest by RT-PCR using 40 cycles. In this case, a positive control tissue should be included to be sure that the probe is intact. Similarly, a positive control probe would be one that detects a good band on Northern blots of the tissue of interest. Immunohistochemistry for the corresponding protein may constitute an additional positive control, but may be negative in spite of positive ISH if the protein or peptide is not stored, as with rapidly secreted peptide hormones (Höfler *et al.* 1988).

However, each probe may require slightly different conditions to optimize the experimental protocol, so that the best negative control for the non-specific binding of the probe itself would be the sense or scrambled sequence probes.

Evaluation of probe quality and troubleshooting

To be sure that a probe of the expected molecular size has been labelled and has not been degraded, an aliquot of $\sim 10^5$ dpm should be run on a sequencing gel including radiolabelled DNA standards. cRNA and oligonucleotide bands should be easily visible as single bands of the expected molecular size. Random-primed cDNAs should range between 400 and 600 bps in length.

If probe synthesis fails ($< 10^7$ dpm/μg) or probe is degraded (as may occur if alkaline hydrolysis is carried out for more than 10 min or as a result of RNase contamination), troubleshooting is recommended as follows.

1. Recheck the integrity of the template cDNA or oligonucleotide prior to repeating synthesis of the probe on an ethidium bromide gel.

2. Be sure that the radiolabelled NTPs or dNTPs are less than two weeks old.

3. Use fresh enzyme, buffers, DTT, and nuclease-free water for probe synthesis.

4. Be sure that yeast tRNA is added as a carrier prior to ethanol precipitation.

In summary, the preparation of labelled probe is one of the critical determinants of the outcome of an ISH experiment. It is always wise to be sure that a labelled probe is of high specific activity and that it is intact. Time spent on probe design and synthesis is usually well spent.

References

Ausubel, F.M., Brent, R., Kingston, R.E., Moore, D.D., Smith, J.A., Seidman, J.G., and Struhl, K. (1987). *Current protocols in molecular biology*. Greene Publishing Associates and Wiley-Interscience, New York.

Baskin, D.G. and Stahl, W.L. (1993). Fundamentals of quantitative autoradiography by computer densitometry for *in situ* hybridization, with emphasis on ^{33}P. *J. Histochem. Cytochem.*, **41**, 1767–76.

Biroc, S.L., Murphy-Erdosh, C., Fisher, J.M., and Payan, D.G. (1993). THe use of ^{33}P-labeled oligonucleotides for *in situ* hybridization of vertebrate embryo frozen sections. *Bio techniques*, **15**, 250–4.

Black, M., Carey, F.A., Farquharson, M.A., Murray, G.D., and McNicol, A.M. (1993). Expression of the pro-opiomelanocortin gene in lung neuroendocrine tumours: *in situ* hybridization and immunohistochemical studies. *J. Pathol.*, **169**, 329–34.

Chantratita, W., Henchal, E.A., and Yoosook, C. (1989). Rapid detection of herpes simplex virus DNA by *in situ* hybridization with photobiotin-labelled double-stranded DNA probes. *Mol. Cell. Probes*, **3**, 363–73.

Davis, L.G., Dibner, M.D., and Battey, J.F. (1986). *Basic methods in molecular biology*. Elsevier, New York.

Denny, P., Hamid, Q., Krause, J.E., Polak, J.M., and Legon, S. (1988). Oligoribo-probes: tools for *in situ* hybridization. *Histochemistry*, **89**, 481–3.

Dirks, R.W., van Gijlswijk, R.P., Vooijs, M.A., Smit, A.B., Bogerd, J., van Minnen, J., Raap, A.K., and van der Ploeg, M. (1991). 3'-end fluorochromized and haptenized oligonucleotides as *in situ* hybridization probes for multiple, simultaneous RNA detection. *Exp. Cell. Res.*, **194**, 310–15.

Eisenstein, B.I. (1990). The polymerase chain reaction: a new method of using molecular genetics for medical diagnosis. *N. Engl. J. Med.*, **322**, 178–83.

Eldridge, J., Zehner, Z., and Paterson, B.M. (1985). Nucleotide sequence of the chicken cardiac alpha actin gene: absence of strong homologies in the promoter and 3'-untranslated regions with the skeletal alpha actin sequence. *Gene*, **36**, 55–63.

Erlich, H.A., Gelfand, D., and Sninsky, J.J. (1991). Recent advances in the polymerase chain reaction. *Science*, **252**, 1643–51.

Evans, M.R. and Read, C.A. (1992). ^{32}P, ^{33}P and ^{35}S: selecting a label for nucleic acid analysis. *Nature*, **358**, 520–1.

Forster, A.C., McInnes, J.L., Skingle, D.C., and Symons, R.H. (1985). Non-radioactive hybridization probes prepared by the chemical labelling of DNA and RNA with a novel reagent, photobiotin. *Nucl. Acids Res.* **13**, 745–61.

Höfler, H., Delellis, R.A., and Wolfe, H.J. (1988). *In situ* hybridization and Immunohistochemistry. In: *Advances in immunohistochemistry*, (ed. R.A. DeLellis), pp. 47–66. Raven Press, New York.

Humpel, C., Lindqvist, E., and Olson, L. (1993). Detection of nerve growth factor mRNA in rodent salivary glands with digoxigenin- and ^{33}P-labeled oligonucleotides: effects of castration and sympathectomy. *J. Histochem. Cytochem.*, **41**, 703–8.

Johnston, D., Hatzis, D., and Sunday, M.E. (1998). Expression of v-Ha-*ras* driven by the calcitonin/calcitonin gene-related peptide promoter: a novel transgenic murine model for medullary thyroid carcinoma. *Oncogene*, **16**, 167–77.

Jostarndt, K., Puntschart, A., Hoppeler, H., and Billeter, R. (1994). The use of ^{33}P-labelled riboprobes for *in situ* hybridizations; localization of myosin alkali light-chain mRNAs in adult human skeletal muscle. *Histochem. J.*, **26**, 32–40

Khan, A.M. and Wright, P.J. Detection of flavivirus RNA in infected cells using photobiotin-labelled hybridization probes. *J. Virol. Meth.*, **15**, 121–30.

Komminoth, P. (1992). Digoxigenin as an alternative probe labeling for *in situ* hybridization. *Diagn. Mol. Pathol.*, **1**, 142–50.

Long, A.A., Mueller, J., Andre-Schwartz, J., Barrett, K.J., Schwartz, R., and Wolfe, H. (1992). High-specificity *in situ* hybridization. Methods and application. *Diagn. Mol. Pathol.* **1**, 45–57.

McInnes, J.L., Forster, A.C., Skingle, D.C., and Symons, R.H. (1990). Preparation and uses of photobiotin. *Meth. Enzymol.*, **184**, 588–600.

McLaughlin, S.K. and Margolskee, R.F. (1993). [33]P is preferable to ^{35}S for labeling probes used in *in situ* hybridization. *Bio techniques*, **15**, 506–11.

Miyajima, N., Horiuchi, R., Shibuya, Y., Fukushige, S., Matsubara, K., Toyoshima, K., and Yamamoto, T. (1989). Two erbA homologs encoding proteins with different T3 binding capacities are transcribed from opposite DNA strands of the same genetic locus. *Cell*, **57**, 31–9.

Niedobitek, G., Finn, T., Herbst, H., and Stein, H. (1989). Detection of viral genomes in the liver by *in situ* hybridization using [35]S-, bromodeoxyuridine-, and biotin-labeled probes. *Am. J. Pathol.*, **134**, 633–9.

Pagani, A., Cerrato, M., and Bussolati, G. (1993). Nonspecific *in situ* hybridization reaction in neuroendocrine cells and tumors of the gastrointestinal tract using oligonucleotide probes. *Diagn. Mol. Pathol.*, **2**, 125–30.

Pang, M. and Baum, L.G. (1993). Application of nonistopic RNA *in situ* hybridization to detect endogenous gene expression in pathologic specimens. *Diagn. Mol. Pathol.*, **2**, 277–82.

Shapiro, J. (1981). *Radiation protection: a guide for scientists and physicians*. 2nd edn. Harvard University Press, Cambridge.

Singer, R.H. and Ward, D.C. (1982). Actin gene expression visualized in chicken muscle tissue culture by using *in situ* hybridization with a biotinylated nucleotide analog. *Proc. Natl. Acad. Sci. USA*, **79**, 7331–5.

Spindel, E.R., Sunday, M.E., Höfler, H., Wolfe, H.J., Habener, J.F. and Chin, W.W. Transient elevation of mRNAs encoding gastrin-releasing peptide (GRP), a putative pulmonary growth factor, in human fetal lung. *J. Clin. Invest.*, **80**, 1172–9.

Steel, J.H., Hamid, Q., van Noorden, S., Jones, P., Denny, P., Burrin, J., Legon, S., Bloom, S.R., and Polak, J.M. (1988). Combined use of *in situ* hybridization and immunohistochemistry for the investigation of prolactin gene expression in immature, pubertal, pregnant, lactating and ovariectomized rats. *Histochemistry*, **89**, 75–80.

Sunday, M.E. (1991). Cell-specific localization of neuropeptide gene expression: gastrin-releasing peptide (GRP; mammalian bombesin). *Meth. Neurosci.*, **5**, 123–36.

Sunday, M.E., Wolfe, H.J., Roos, B.A., Chin, W.W., and Spindel, E.R. (1988). Gastrin-releasing peptide gene expression in developing, hyperplastic, and neoplastic human thyroidal C-cells. *Endocrinology*, **122**, 1551–8.

Sunday, M.E., Choi, N., Spindel, E.R., Chin, W.W., and Mark, E. (1991). Gastrin-releasing peptide gene expression in small cell and large cell undifferentiated lung carcinomas. *Hum. Pathol.*, **22**, 1030–9.

van den Brink, W., van der Loos, C., Volkers, H., Lauwen, R., van den Berg, F., Houthoff, H.J., and Das, P.K. (1990). Combined beta-galactosidase and immunogold/silver staining for immunohistochemistry and DNA *in situ* hybridization. *J. Histochem. Cytochem.*, **38**, 325–9.

Wada, E., Battey, J., and Wray, S. (1993). Bombesin receptor gene expression in rat embryos: transient GRP-R gene expression in the posterior pituitary. *Mol. Cell. Neurosci.*, **4**, 13–24.

Wang, D. and Cutz, E. (1994). Simultaneous detection of messenger ribonucleic acids for bombesin/gastrin-releasing peptide and its receptor in rat brain by non-radiolabeled double *in situ* hybridization. *Lab. Invest.*, **70**, 775–80.

Yamada, S., Takahashi, M., Hara, M., Sano, T., Aiba, T., Shishiba, Y., Suzuki, T., and Asa, S.L. (1994). Growth hormone and prolactin gene expression in human densely and sparsely granulated somatotroph adenomas by *in situ* hybridization and digoxigenin-labeled probes. *Diagn. Mol. Pathol.*, **3**, 46–52.

3

The preparation of non-radioisotopic hybridization probes

CHRISTOPHER J. BAKKENIST and JAMES O'D. McGEE

The detection of specific nucleic acid sequences in DNA or RNA, which have been biochemically purified and immobilized on a membrane, either directly, or by transfer following electrophoretic fractionation, is one of the most prevalent methodologies used in molecular biology. The sequences of interest are detected on the membrane by hybridization to a labelled nucleic acid probe. The molecules most commonly used to label probes are radionuclides, which may be detected indirectly using autoradiography, and radionuclides remain the most resilient labels available. The purpose of *in situ* hybridization is the detection of specific nucleic acid sequences in intact cells, such as *Drosophila* oocytes, or within tissue sections, such as human biopsies, and requires the presence of the DNA or RNA sequence of interest to be correlated with microscopic morphology. This chapter describes, with special emphasis on *in situ* hybridization, the preparation of nucleic acid probes using the principal non-radioactive labels that have been developed.

Non-radioisotopic label molecules

Biotin

Many different molecules have been used as probe labels but the most widely employed are biotin (Dale *et al*. 1973) and digoxigenin (Syvanen *et al*. 1985). Analogues of dUTP, UTP, dATP, and ATP that contain a biotin molecule covalently linked to the C-5 position of the pyrimidine ring through a linker arm are efficient substrates for several polymerases *in vitro* (Table 3.1). Synthesized polynucleotides containing low levels of conjugated biotin show similar hybridization characteristics to their native counterparts. As the degree of biotin-labelled nucleotide incorporated into the probe increases the thermal stability (melting temperature, T_m) of the probe–target sequence hybrid decreases slightly. This can be determined empirically.

The simplest detection systems for biotin (and most other labels) are based on a single step involving an antibody conjugated directly to an indicator enzyme

Table 3.1 Enzymatic labelling of probes

Label	Enzyme	Probe
x-dUTO: x can be biotin digoxigenin; fluorescein rhodamine; coumarin **x-dATP:** x can be biotin	DNA polymerase I; Klenow fragment; Taq DNA polymerase; T7 DNA polymerase; reverse transcriptase	Double-stranded DNA Single-stranded DNA
x-UTP: x can be biotin; digoxigenin; fluorescein; rhodamine; coumarin **x-dATP:** x can be biotin	SP6, T3, and T7 RNA, polymerases	Single-stranded RNA
x-ddUTP or dUTP: x can be biotin; digoxigenin; fluorescein	Terminal transferase	3'-ends of DNA fragments; oligonucleotides

or fluorescence marker (Langer *et al.* 1981). Incubation of the enzyme-coupled antibody with the enzyme substrate produces stable, coloured reaction products which can be visualized using conventional microscopy. Alkaline phosphatase is the enzyme most commonly used as an indicator in the reporter complex. The positive signals are developed by incubation with BCIP (5-bromo-4-chloro-3-indolyl phosphate) and the chromogenic reagent NBT (nitroblue tetrazolium). Horseradish peroxidase is also widely used and is detected by using hydrogen peroxidase and DAB (diamonobenzidine) or other compounds. Fluorescent dyes produce a signal of higher resolution than enzymatic detection methods. Fluorescent techniques are not readily applicable to routine laboratory situations, however, since the equipment required for fluorescence microscopy is expensive and paraffin-embedded tissue auto-fluoresces.

Non-immunological detection in which the enzyme or fluorescent dye is coupled to avidin or streptavidin is also possible. Both avidin and streptavidin have extremely high binding affinities for biotin ($K_d = 10^{-15}$ for the binding of these molecules, whereas the maximum binding affinity of an antibody for an antigen is $K_d = 10^{-12}$). Avidin, however, a glycoprotein, binds to lectins and negatively charged biomolecules (such as DNA) under certain conditions, which can result in an increased non-specific background signal. Streptavidin has therefore generally superseded avidin in the reporter molecule as it is not glycosylated and has higher specificity.

Signal amplification can be achieved either by antibody layering techniques or by increasing the number of enzyme molecules bound to each reporter molecule. The two methods of antibody and enzyme enhancement are combined in methods based on the avidin biotintylated enzyme reporter complex. In one method avidin is used as a bridge between the primary target (biotinylated DNA) and detectors (biotinylated enzymes). Alternatively a pre-formed complex of avidin and biotinylated enzyme, which is biotin-binding dominant, is used to detect the biotin-labelled probe. Unfortunately, as the sensitivity is increased the background is also increased as side reactions will be generated, since biotin itself is found in almost all natural materials. Signal amplification techniques are discussed in detail in Chapters 9 and 10.

Digoxigenin

Digoxigenin is of plant origin (extracted from *Digitalis* plants) and therefore results in low, non-specific staining due to endogenous products. The molecule can be linked to uridine nucleotides at the 5 position in the pyrimidine ring (Boehringer Mannheim) and the resultant nucleotide analogues function as efficient substrates for several DNA-modifying enzymes. Following signal amplification and immunological detection, digoxigenin-labelled probes are as sensitive as biotin-labelled probes (Herrington *et al.* 1989, 1991). Signal amplification may be achieved in the following manner; a monoclonal antibody to digoxigenin is linked via a biotinylated rabbit anti-mouse immunoglobulin to avidin alkaline phosphatase.

Fluorochromes

The first available flurorochrome-labelled nucleotides were dideoxynuleotides which were produced for non-radioactive DNA sequencing. Fluorescein- (yellow-green), rhodamine- (red), and coumarine- (blue) labelled dUTPs are now commercially available and can be enzymatically incorporated into probes (Amersham International). These labels may be detected directly by fluorescence microscopy or indirectly by immunological techniques. Visual mapping by fluorescent *in situ* hybridization (FISH) is the most direct approach for the localization of genomic clones to a chromosome. The ability to detect several hybridization signals simultaneously by using fluorescent labels with different colours has allowed the relative positioning of different clones and gene orientation to be determined by FISH (Heiskanen *et al.* 1996). Ordering of clones on metaphase chromosomes requires that the differentially labelled probes are separated by at least 1 Mb (Trask *et al.* 1991). In interphase nuclei, however, the chromatin is less condensed than in metaphase chromosomes, allowing the visual mapping of the genomic distance between probes over a range of 25 kb to at least 250 kb (Trask *et al.* 1989). The ease of preparation of the hybridization target has made FISH to inter- phase nuclei readily amenable to studies of cytogenetic disorders. Fluorescein has also been used to label anti-mouse and anti-rabbit immunoglobulins in order to permit the detection of these antibodies using fluorescence.

Preparation of labelled probes

There are two major approaches to probe labelling. These are labelling by enzymatic modification and labelling by chemical modification.

Labelling by enzymatic modification

Nick translation

Nick translation (Rigby *et al.* 1977) is probably the most widely employed method for labelling hybridization probes used to detect DNA sequences. In the procedure, double-stranded DNA is incubated with bovine pancreatic deoxyribonuclease I (DNase I) and *E. coli* DNA polymerase I (Pol I) in the presence of three unlabelled deoxyribonucleoside triphosphates, the fourth labelled deoxyribonucleoside triphosphate, and magnesium ions. The DNA may be either inserted probe sequences removed from a vector by restriction digestion or the entire recombinant clone (either plasmid or phage). In the latter case, the possibility of hybridization of the native vector must be excluded using the appropriate negative control.

DNase I is an endonuclease that hydrolyses double-stranded and single-stranded DNA into a complex mixture of oligonuleotides and nucleotides with 5'-phosphate termini. In the presence of Mg^{2+}, however, DNase I introduces single-stranded nicks into double-stranded DNA at random. Pol I is the *E. coli* DNA polymerase responsible for the repair of the bacterial chromosome. The holoenzyme is a 5'–3' DNA polymerase with both a 5'–3' exonuclease and a 3'–5' 'proof-reading' exonuclease. Pol I can therefore initiate DNA synthesis at a single-stranded nick on a double-stranded DNA template. Thus, in the nick translation reaction, DNase I functions to produce 'priming' sites for Pol I, which can subsequently replace deoxyribonucleotides from the nicked strand in a 5'–3' direction using the complementary strand of the DNA as a template. This polymerization proceeds until the processivity of the enzyme is exhausted, and results in the incorporation of a labelled deoxyribonucleotide into the double-stranded DNA in place of one of the original nucleotides. Theoretically, the double-stranded DNA is uniformly labelled by the procedure, since the DNase I introduces nicks into both strands of the DNA in a random fashion. Following heat denaturation the probe consists of a pool of labelled, overlapping, single-stranded fragments of varying length, which are cumulatively representative of the original DNA.

During the hybridization of a nick-translated probe it is possible that the overlapping sequences at the ends of the fragments could anneal together to produce a probe network which could function to amplify the target sequence *in vitro*. This probe networking potential may make probes produced by nick translation the most suitable for the achievement of high sensitivity in *in situ* hybridization, since the length of the probe fragments can be most highly controlled using this method (Gerhard *et al.* 1981). It may also explain why many workers find probes prepared from recombinant clones are more sensitive than those prepared from insert sequences alone, since fragments containing the vector and insert sequences will direct the vector probe fragments to the hybridization site.

The structure of a probe generated by the nick translation reaction frequently has to be optimized in order to obtain the highest sensitivity. Ideally, following denaturation, the fragment lengths should be in a small range and each should be uniformly labelled. Probe lengths of 50–400 bp are optimal for *in situ* hybridization, since the probe must be able to penetrate the tissue. The average length of the labelled probe fragments can be varied by titrating the concentration of DNase I and therefore the number of nicks generated in the reaction. The frequency at which the label is incorporated into the probe can be controlled by varying the concentration of Pol I and that of the labelled nucleotide used in the reaction. The length of the incubation time should also be optimized. Typically, the quality of the probe produced by an established set of reaction conditions is a reflection on the purity of the DNA used in the reaction. Different contaminants present in DNA preparations from distinct sources may inhibit one of the enzyme activities required for nick translation, thereby altering their sensitive balance. In order to avoid performing continuous series of optimization reactions, the use of extremely pure DNA and nick translation reagents is essential.

Random-primed labelling

Random-primed labelling (Feinberg and Vogelstein 1983) is based on the indiscriminate priming of DNA synthesis on denatured DNA by hexamer oligonucleotides of heterogeneous sequence (Random hexamers). Double-stranded, supercoiled DNA molecules to be labelled by this procedure must be linearized prior to denaturation in order to prevent the rapid reannealing of the single-stranded template DNA. More typically, however, the probe insert sequences are removed from vector sequences by restriction digestion prior to labelling. Following heat denaturation the single-stranded DNA is incubated in the presence of three unlabelled deoxyribonucleoside triphosphates, the fourth labelled deoxyribonucleoside triphosphate, random hexamers, and the Klenow fragment of *E. coli* DNA polymerase I. The Klenow fragment of *E. coli* DNA polymerase I retains the DNA polymerase activity and the 3′–5′ exonuclease but lacks the 5′–3′ exonuclease. This fragment synthesizes DNA on the single-stranded DNA template primed by the free 3′-hydroxyl group of an annealed random hexamer. DNA synthesis proceeds until the enzyme reaches a second annealed random hexamer which has served to 'prime' DNA synthesis or exhausts its processivity, and the labelled deoxyribonucleotide is incorporated into the DNA in the appropriate complementary fashion.

Since the priming of DNA synthesis is indiscriminate, and both strands of the DNA serve as templates, the probe produced by random labelling consists of a pool of overlapping single-stranded fragments of varying length, which are again theoretically representative of the original DNA following heat denaturation. Probes generated by random priming are, however, composed of a higher proportion of short fragments than nick translated probes, which can lead to a higher non-specific background staining. The length of the labelled strands can be controlled by varying the ratio of the primer to template, but this must be determined empirically because of the non-random sequence of DNA. Any regions of secondary structure in the single-stranded template used for random-primed labelling tend to be underrepresented in the probe, and it inevitably contains both labelled (synthesized) and non-labelled single-stranded DNA. Thus, only a maximum of half of the final hybridized probe is labelled and this results in random-primed probes having a lower sensitivity than nick translated probes. Any signal amplification produced by networking potential is also reduced by half. A greater incorporation of label can be achieved by random-primed labelling than by nick translation, however, and the method is also more reliable and more reproducible. This reproducibility is a result of both the relative simplicity of the enzyme activities required for random-primed labelling when compared with those required for nick translation, and the resilience of the Klenow fragment to inhibition by contaminants in DNA preparations. Indeed, random-primed probes can be synthesized in the presence of agarose, which is a potent inhibitor of many DNA-modifying enzymes. Random-primed labelling is therefore particularly useful for DNA samples that are not of the highest purity, such as those typically purified from agarose gels, and for short DNA fragments, which do not label well by nick translation.

Probe generation by the polymerase chain reaction

The polymerase chain reaction (PCR) is an *in vitro* method for the exponential amplification of a specific DNA fragment from a small amount of template. Amplification is performed between two oligonucleotide primers using a thermostable DNA polymerase and thermal cycling between DNA denaturation, oligonucleotide annealing, and DNA synthesis temperatures. By replacing a deoxyribonucleoside triphosphate with a labelled analogue in the PCR reaction mixture, label can be incorporated into the amplified DNA product at a density superior to that which can be obtained by either nick translation or random-primed probe synthesis (Lichter *et al.* 1990). The density of the label incorporated into the probe can be varied by replacing a proportion of the nucleotide analogue with the corresponding unlabelled nucleotide. Equivalent molarities of all four nucleotides must be maintained in the PCR reaction mixture in order to ensure the synthesis of full-length products.

PCR is the method of choice for probe preparation when the amount of DNA available for probe preparation is low, such as tumour DNA or microdissected chromosome bands. It is also of use when probes must be contrived from templates where the preparation of recombinant clones would be extremely costly and cannot be justified. This is the case when the template is derived from hybrid cell lines (Lichter *et al.* 1990) or yeast artificial chromosomes (Breen *et al.* 1992).

Since the PCR reaction is capable of amplifying a single molecule of DNA, precautions must be taken to guard against contamination of the reaction mixtures with exogenous DNA. Where possible, the identity of the amplified probe should always be confirmed by direct sequencing or restriction fragment mapping. Towards this end, DNA fragments amplified from a complex or mixed template should be labelled in a second round of PCR amplification using the resolved target sequence as the template. The purification of the amplified product from the primary PCR removes DNA fragments produced non-specifically during the initial cycles of the PCR. Alternatively, if the amplified fragment is large, it can be amplified using the four unlabelled deoxribonucleoside triphospates and then labelled by either nick translation or random-primed labelling.

A probe prepared using PCR consists of two complementary labelled single strands each of which is the length of the amplified product; typically 180 bp to 2 bp. It can therefore be necessary to incubate the double-stranded, amplified DNA product with DNase I in order to obtain fragments of the appropriate size for *in situ* hybridization prior to use.

It is possible to add DNA sequences that are not complementary to the template DNA at the 5'-end of the oligonucleotide primers used in a PCR reaction. These non-complementary sequences become incorporated in the amplified DNA sequence. A DNA fragment can therefore be amplified between oligonucleotides, one of which has a promoter for a bacteriophage RNA polymerase at its 5'-end, in order to create a target that can be transcribed by the RNA polymerase. In this manner a labelled RNA transcript can be produced without having to resort to subcloning the DNA segment into a vector with a bacteriophage RNA polymerase promoter (Schowalter and Sommer, 1989).

Primed *in situ* labelling of DNA (PRINS) and *in situ* PCR

The PRINS technique is based on the *in situ* synthesis of non-radioisotopic hybridization probes (Koch *et al.* 1989). Unlabelled, denatured double-stranded DNA fragments (or, more recently, unlabelled synthetic oligonucleotide primers) produced by PCR, or purified from recombinant clones, are annealed in a sequence-specific fashion to fixed chromosome preparations. This DNA then serves as a primer for chain elongation *in situ*, catalysed by a DNA polymerase (Pol I, Klenow fragment or Taq DNA polymerase). If biotin-labelled nucleotides are used as a substrate for chain elongation the hybridization site becomes labelled with biotin. The biotin is subsequently detected using fluorescein-labelled avidin and is visualized using fluorescence microscopy. This procedure has been used for the cytogenetic localization of high copy number, chromosome-specific, tandem repeat sequences, including centromeric, telomeric, and satellite sequences (Koch *et al.* 1991). The detection of single copy sequences remains problematic using the PRINS technique.

The PRINS procedure has also been used to detect RNA *in situ* (Mogensen *et al.* 1991). In the reaction, unlabelled oligonucleotide primers were annealed to intracellular RNA and subsequent chain elongation catalysed by reverse transcriptase. Biotin labelled nucleotides were incorporated into the hybridization probe *in situ* and detected as above.

The *in situ* synthesis of non-radioisotopic hybridization probes has also been accomplished using Taq DNA polymerase and thermal cycling between DNA denaturation, oligonucleotide annealing, and DNA synthesis temperatures in order to detect single copy sequences. *In situ* PCR, refers to the exponential amplification of cellular DNA sequences between two oligonucleotides with concurrent incorporation of a labelled nucleotide (a labelled oligonucleotide can also be used). *In situ* reverse transcriptase PCR (RT-PCR) for the amplification of mRNA sequences has also been performed. In this technique, cDNA is synthesized by reverse transcriptase and then amplified as for *in situ* PCR. The labelled products produced in these reactions are detected using the standard detection techniques. The detection of a signal in a cell following *in situ* PCR only proves that a single oligonucleotide annealed to a sequence of DNA in that cell (at the stringency determined by the reaction conditions) and served as a primer to initiate DNA synthesis. Diffusion of the amplified DNA fragments out of the cells of origin is also a current problem with the technique. Theoretically, *in situ* endoreplication to produce very short regions of 'polytene chromosomes', which could be visualized following the incorporation of a labelled nucleotide using fluorescence microscopy, confined in the nucleus or preferably on a chromosome, would be a superior technique.

Single-stranded DNA probes

Single-stranded DNA probes can be obtained from sequences cloned into bacteriophage M13 or phagemids activated by phage superinfection. The advantage of single-stranded DNA probes (and riboprobes) is that there are no complementary sequences to the probe present in the hybridization reaction except for the cellular target. Other probes are used following the heat denaturation of two complementary DNA strands, and these strands can reanneal in the hybridization solution, reducing the effective concentration of probe available. Since these single-stranded DNA probes are strand specific they can be used for the localization of RNA.

Single-stranded probes labelled with nucleotide analogues may be prepared using the Klenow fragment or T7 DNA polymerase. DNA synthesis is primed by a sequence-specific oligonucleotide annealed to the single-stranded phage DNA template. Prior to the DNA synthesis reaction, the single-stranded phage may be linearized with a restriction enzyme if an oligonucleotide encoding a restriction enzyme site is annealed to its complementary sequence. If this restriction enzyme site is in either the inserted DNA or the polylinker downstream of the insert then the length of the probe can be defined.

In order to purify the single-stranded probe, the double-stranded DNA synthesized is denatured using sodium hydroxide. This DNA mixture is then resolved by electrophoresis through an alkaline agarose gel. Following its visualization using ethidium bromide, the single-stranded probe can be gel purified by any conventional methodology. If the single-stranded phage DNA was not linearized prior to the labelling reaction, the size of the probe fragments can be selected in the gel. Since single-stranded DNA does not intercalate ethidium bromide efficiently, small amounts of short probes may not stain well. Single-stranded DNA probes prepared in this fashion are highly specific and produce very little background staining. Their advantage over single-stranded RNA probes is the relative ease with which they may be prepared and used owing to their greater stability than riboprobes.

Single-stranded DNA probes can be prepared by a primer extension mechanism using the Klenow fragment or T7 DNA polymerase from linearized, denatured, double-stranded DNA templates. The efficiency of the labelling reaction on denatured double-stranded DNA templates is low in comparison with that on single-stranded DNA templates because of the tendency of the former to reanneal.

Single-stranded DNA probes can also be prepared by asymmetric PCR in which the amplification oligonucleotides are added in a molar ratio of 100:1. The relative concentrations of the oligonucleotides and target required must be determined empirically. PCR is performed as described above for double-stranded probe preparation and proceeds by the same mechanism for the initial cycles, in order to amplify a specific target sequence exponentially. One of the oligonucleotides is then exhausted and the Taq polymerase is then only able to amplify one of the target strands linearly. These probes are used directly following denaturation and are therefore never homogeneous for the single strand, which has been amplified in excess.

In vitro transcription

Single-stranded RNA probes (riboprobes) are used extensively for the highly specific and sensitive detection of mRNA. Riboprobes are generated by *in vitro* transcription from linearized recombinant cDNA clones (or PCR-amplified DNA fragments, as discussed earlier) which contain RNA polymerase promoters downstream of the sense cDNA strand. The three most commonly used RNA polymerases are those encoded by the T3, T7, and SP6 bacteriophage (see Chapter 2). Riboprobes are prepared by incubating the RNA polymerase with template DNA in the presence of three unlabelled ribonucleoside triphosphates and the fourth labelled ribonucleoside triphosphate. The RNA polymerase binds its specific promoter in the double-stranded DNA target and initiates RNA synthesis using the sense cDNA strand as a template. RNA polymerization proceeds until the end of the linearized template is reached. It is therefore possible to control the length of a riboprobe by restriction digestion of the cDNA. Alternatively, riboprobes representing the full-length transcript can be reduced to the desired length by controlled alkaline lysis. Numerous RNA molecules are transcribed from each double-stranded DNA template. Prior to use the DNA present in the probe is degraded using DNase I in order to obviate any background that could be produced by non-specific, tissue-recombinant DNA clone–riboprobe complexes.

The incorporation of biotin-labelled UTP into a riboprobe by SP6 RNA polymerase is very low and the use of T3 and T7 RNA polymerases with this nucleotide analogue is therefore favoured. Alternatively, an allylamine de-rivative of UTP can be incorporated into the transcript by SP6 RNA polymerase and subsequently biotinylated chemically.

Digoxigenin also inhibits all three RNA polymerases in a dose-dependent manner (Höltke and Kessler 1990). The concentration of digoxigenin nucleo-tide analogue in the reaction mixture must therefore be optimized in order to achieve the maximum incorporation of the label into the riboprobe. The best results are obtained when equivalent molarities of all four nucleotides are maintained in the reaction and any reduction in the concentration of the nucleotide analogue should be compensated for with unlabelled nucleotide (Heer *et al.* 1994).

RNA–RNA hybrids are more stable than RNA–DNA hybrids, and the de-tection of RNA using riboprobes under conditions that obviate riboprobe–DNA binding is therefore possible. Background, non-specific staining can be reduced by degradation of single-stranded RNA with RNase following hybridization, since RNA–RNA hybrids are resistant to digestion by this enzyme. Since non-specific RNA binding by the riboprobe can occur if the stringency used is too low, sense RNA riboprobes are a useful negative control for the localization of specific a mRNA species by *in situ* hybrid-ization. These can readily be prepared from recombinant cDNA clones that contain different RNA polymerase promoters either side of the insert. Failing this, the cDNA insert must be cloned into the vector in both orientations.

3′-End labelling using terminal transferase

Terminal deoxyribonucleotidyl transferase (terminal transferase) catalyses the polmerization of deoxyribonucleoside triphospates into polynucleotides on a 3′-hydroxyl group at the end of either double-stranded or single-stranded DNA (including oligonucleotides). It is the only enzyme known that poly-merizes nucleotides in a template-independent fashion. This activity can be used to synthesize labelled homopolymeric tails using a nucleotide analogue substrate on an unlabelled specific target sequence. Target DNA sequences are typically 100–200 bp fragments. The unlabelled target sequence serves as a homogeneous hybridization probe and has the same T_m as native DNA of the same length and GC content, and probes prepared in this way can be advantageous if T_m is critical. The hybridization of probes labelled by this method can be subject to a high background noise since the homopolymeric tail synthesized is not specific for the sequence of interest. Probes labelled with terminal transferase do not have wide applications.

Table 3.2 Advantages and disadvantages of enzymatic methods for preparing non-isotopic probes

Labelling method	Advantages	Disadvantages
Double-stranded DNA probes	1. Choice of labelling methods available 2. Amplification of signal by networking 3. Hybridization temperature less critical	1. Probe denaturation required 2. Reannealing in hybridization reaction 3. Purification of insert can be necessary to remove background
Nick translation Length of probe	1. Very high sensitivity 2. Activities sensitive to inhibitors and highly controllable	1. Balance of enzyme 2. Fragments in small range
Random-primed labelling	1. Robustness of technique 2. Very high levels of label incorporation can be achieved 3. High sensitivity	1. Length of probe fragments less controllable, resulting in more background 2. Less networking potential 3. At least 50% of final probe is unlabelled
PCR-generated probes	1. No subcloning required 2. Probes can be prepared from subnanogram quantities of complex/mixed targets	1. Possible contamination leading to background or even incorrect fragment amplification 2. DNase I treatment of probe may be necessary 3. Less networking potential
PRINS and *in situ* PCR	1. Speed of technique	1. Possible incorrect annealing of primers leading to false positives 2. Very low specificity
Single-stranded probes	1. High specificity 2. No reannealing in hybridization reaction 3. No denaturation required	1. No networking potential 2. Complicated to prepare
Single-stranded DNA probes		1. Directional subcloning into phage or phagemid required
Riboprobes	1. High stability of RNA–RNA 2. Post-hybridization RNase treatment removes non-hybridized probe	1. Narrow optimum hybridization temperature 2. Possible probe degradation by RNase 3. Subcloning into dual promoter vector required

Labelling by chemical modification

Photoactivation for labelling

A photoreactive biotin can be used to biotinylate DNA, RNA, and protein randomly (Forster *et al.* 1985). The analogue consists of biotin linked via a positively charged linker arm to the photoactive group. The molecule is attracted to DNA and RNA by the ionic interaction between the positively charged linker arm and phosphate groups in the nucleic acid chains. Following photoactivation the analogue cross-links to the aromatic bases of nucleic acids.

Biotin probes prepared by photoactivation are not as sensitive as those prepared enzymatically because of the relatively low level of incorporation of the biotinyl residues. Hybridizations performed with these probes also have higher non-specific background noise because any contaminants in the nucleic acid preparation are biotinylated during the procedure, and non-specific tissue are bound by the positively charged unbound biotin analogue.

Bisulfite modifications

Cytidine residues can be modified by transamination with sodium bisulfite and ethylenediamine. The result is the introduction of amino groups on the pyrimidine ring. Fluorescent molecules can be coupled to these amino groups on the cytidine molecules in either RNA or DNA (Draper 1984). A modification procedure for the binding of activated digoxigenin to the amino groups is available (Boehringer Mannheim) and biotin ester can also be reacted with the amino groups (Viscidi *et al.* 1986).

As mentioned above, the incorporation of biotin-labelled UTP into RNA by SP6 RNA polymerase is very low. Allylamine-labelled UTP is incorporated efficiently into RNA by the enzyme. The analogue incorporated into the RNA can be labelled following synthesis, by reaction with biotin ester. Similarly, allylamine-modified nucleotides can be incorporated by all the enzyme techniques used to prepare labelled probes, and the nucleic acids synthesized can be subsequently labelled. Since the allylamine modification is very small, these analogues are more efficient substrates for the enzymes than the large biotin-, digoxigenin-, and fluorescently labelled nucleotide analogues. Biotinylation with biotin ester is highly controllable and probes can be prepared by this two-step procedure in a highly reproducible fashion.

Chemical labelling of oligonucleotides at their 5′-termini

An oligonucleotide primer can be used as a homogeneous probe for *in situ* hybridization. These probes have several advantages over those described above. No cloning is required to generate an oligonucleotide probe from any deduced nucleic acid or amino sequence and very specific probes can be prepared following homology searches for any related sequences. Oligonucleotides cannot self-hybridize since they are single stranded, and they also show good target penetration. The sensitivity of oligonucleotides is low, however, since their small size limits the amount of label that they can carry, they have no networking potential, and their hybridization is not as stable as that of other probes. Oligonucleotides can be chemically labelled at the 5'-terminus through a linker arm to any of the label molecules discussed above and these labelled molecules can be purchased commercially (Chollet and Kawashima 1985).

Mercuration of nucleic acids

The covalent modification of cytidine and uridine molecules in nucleic acids by mercury introduces anchoring points for several labels. Biotin, fluorescein, and rhodamine have all been bound to DNA and RNA probes in a stable fashion (Hopman *et al.* 1986).

Chemical modification methods are highly reproducible when standardized, but the reactions are complex and some of the reagents are unstable. For chemical labelling methodologies no kits are commercially available. For these reasons, with the exception of the chemical labelling of the 5'-termini of oligonucleotides, the enzymatic preparation of nucleic acid probes is the labelling method of choice for most applications.

Probe purification

After the labelling reaction, probes are purified from unincorporated label prior to use. Rapid Sephadex column chromatography through spun columns prepared using Sephadex G-50 is the most convenient method of probe purification. Unincorporated label is trapped in the column material while the labelled probe is too large to enter the matrix and passes through the column. Conventional column chromatography through the same material yields superior results but is tedious since the fractions containing the probe have to be identified by detection of the label. Unincorporated label can also be eliminated from the probe by ethanol precipitation. If this procedure is performed the probe pellet must be extensively washed using 70% ethanol in order to remove final traces of the label.

Conclusions

Considerable progress has been made in the development of non-radio-isotopic label systems for *in situ* hybridization. The sensitivity of these methods is not yet sufficient, however, to abolish radioactive *in situ* methods completely. Radioactive techniques are still generally required for the routine detection of single copy sequences of 1 kb or less in interphase nuclei. Similarly, radionuclide labels are required for the *in situ* detection of mRNA species that are expressed at low levels and if any quantification of the visualized signals is required.

References

Breen, M., Arveiler, B., Murray, I. *et al.* (1992). YAC mapping by FISH. *Genomics*, **13**, 726–30.

Chollet, A. and Kawashima, E.M. (1985). Biotin-labeled synthetic oligodeoxyribonucleotides. *Nucl. Acids Res.*, **13**, 1529–41.

Dale, R.M.K., Livingston, D.C., and Ward, D.C. (1973). The synthesis and enzymatic polymerization of nucleotides containing mercury. *Proc. Natl. Acad. Sci. USA*, **70**, 2238–42.

Draper, D.E. (1984). Attachment of reporter groups to specific, selected cytidine residues in RNA. *Nucl. Acids Res.*, **12**, 989–1002.

Feinberg, A. and Vogelstein, B. (1983). *Nucl. Acids Res.*, **11**, 5147.

Forster, A.C., McInnes, J.L., Skingle, D.C. *et al.* (1985). Non-radioactive hybridization probes. *Nucl. Acids Res.*, **13**, 745–61.

Gerhard, D.S., Kawasaki, E.S., Bancroft, F.C. *et al.* (1981). Localization of a unique gene by hybridization in situ. *Proc. Natl. Acad. Sci. USA*, **78**, 3755–9.

Heer, A.H., Keyszer, G.M., Gay, R.E. *et al.* (1994). Inhibition of RNA polymerases. *Biotechniques*, **16**, 54–5.

Heiskanen, M., Peltonen, L., and Palotie, A. (1996). Visual mapping by high resolution FISH. *Trends Genet.*, **12**, 379–82.

Herrington, C.S., Burns, J., Graham, A.K., Bhatt, B., and McGee, J.O'D. (1989). Interphase cytogenics. *J. Clin. Pathol.* **42**, 601–6.

Herrington, C.S., Graham, A.K., and McGee, J.O'D. (1991). Interphase cytogenics. *J. Clin. Pathol.*, **44**, 33–8.

Höltke, H.-L. and Kessler, C. (1990). Non-radioactive labeling of RNA transcripts. *Nucl. Acids Res.*, **18**, 5843–51.

Hopman, A.H.N., Wiegant, J., and Van Duijn, P. (1986). A non-radioactive in situ hybridization method. *Nucl. Acids Res.*, **14**, 6471–88.

Koch, J.E., Kolvraa, S., Peterson, K.B. *et al.* (1989). Oligonucleotide-priming methods. *Chromosoma*, **98**, 259–65.

Koch, J.E., Hindkjaer, J., Mogensen, J. *et al.* (1991). An improved method for chromosome-specific labelling. *Genet. Anal. Tech. Appl*, **8**, 171–8.

Langer, P.R., Waldrop, A.A., and Ward, D.C. (1981). Enzymatic synthesis of biotin-labeled polynucleotides. *Proc. Natl. Acad. Sci. USA*, **78**, 6633–7.

Lichter, P., Ledbetter, S.A., Ledbetter, D.H. *et al.* (1990). Fluorescence in situ hybridization. *Proc. Natl. Acad. Sci. USA*, **87**, 6634–8.

Mogensen, J., Kolvraa, S., Hindkjaer, J. *et al.* (1991). Nonradioactive, sequence-specific detection of RNA. *Exp. Cell Res.*, **196**, 92–8.

Rigby, P.W.J., Dieckmann, M., Rhodes, C. *et al.* (1977). Labeling deoxyribonucleic acid. *J. Mol. Biol.*, **113**, 237–51.

Schowalter, D.B. and Sommer, S.S. (1989). The generation of radiolabeled DNA and RNA probes. *Anal. Biochem.* **177**, 90–4.

Syvanen, A.C., Alanen, M., and Soderlund, N. (1985). A complex of single-stranded binding protein and MI3 DNA. *Nucl. Acids Res.*, **13**, 2789–802.

Trask, B.J., Pinkel, D., and van den Enh, G. (1989). The proximity of DNA sequences. *Genomics*, **5**, 710–17.

Trask, B., Massa, H., Kenwrick, S. *et al.* (1991). Mapping of human chromosome Xq28. *Am. J. Hum. Genet.*, **48**, 1–15.

Viscidi, R.P., Connelly, C.J., and Yolken, R.H. (1986). Novel chemical method for the preparation of nucleic acids. *J. Clin. Microbiol.*, **23**, 311–17.

4

Principles and applications of complementary RNA probes

J.H. STEEL, L. GORDON, and J.M. POLAK

Introduction

The use of *in situ* hybridization for the detection of messenger RNA (mRNA) in tissue sections and other types of tissue or cell preparations is widely accepted as being a powerful technique for investigating gene expression at the cellular level. The high specificity and sensitivity of the bond formed between the nucleic acid probe and its target in the tissue section allows the detection of low abundance mRNAs, although there is a detection limit for the technique. In this chapter, the use of complementary RNA (cRNA) probes will be discussed (for a discussion of other types of probes, see Chapters 1–3). The use of RNA probes, otherwise known as riboprobes, for *in situ* hybridization was pioneered by Angerer and colleagues (see Cox *et al.* 1984). Riboprobes are single-stranded molecules produced from a cloned cDNA that has been introduced into a specifically designed plasmid reverse transcription system. The probe remains single stranded and will not form hybrids in solution, so a higher concentration of probe is available for hybridization, giving more intense signals than for DNA probes (see Cox *et al.* 1984). In addition, the cRNA–mRNA hybrids are more stable than corresponding cDNA–mRNA hybrids (Wetmur *et al.* 1981). While cRNA probes may show a greater tendency to bind non-specifically to tissues, this problem can be overcome by the use of RNase in the post-hybridization washes, removing only single-stranded RNA and leaving the newly formed hybrids untouched. RNase contamination during other procedures (while labile target mRNA is present) must be avoided.

Overall, the use of cRNA probes offers considerable advantages over cDNA probes (see Chapters 1 and 2). Recently, *in situ* hybridization methods using oligonucleotide probes have been gaining in popularity. Synthetic oligonucleotides can be custom-made to a desired length, in large quantities, and to high levels of purity, including labelled nucleotides if necessary. They are usually quite short (30–60 bases long) and can be labelled at 3′ and/or 5′ terminal nucleotides, although limitations in the number of labelled nucleotides that can be added by end-labelling restrict the sensitivity of the technique. This may be overcome by using cocktails of oligonucleotides. Oligonucleotides are more easily generated than riboprobes and are just as convenient to use, but riboprobes are likely to provide greater sensitivity, partly because of their increased specific activity. The increased length of a riboprobe compared to an oligoprobe can ensure higher specificity for the target sequence, since a short probe is more likely to bind non-specifically to similar target sequences in non-homologous mRNAs present in the tissue. Synthetic oligonucleotides can be used to construct riboprobes, by inserting oligonucleotides into appropriate vectors to generate cRNA molecules (oligoriboprobes) (Denny *et al.* 1988).

The polymerase chain reaction (PCR) can be used to synthesize riboprobe sequences without insertion of the cDNA sequence into a vector. The PCR reaction normally generates a mixture of double-stranded (sense and anti-sense) sequences, which can be labelled during the PCR reaction and then used directly as a probe, although these could be regarded as cDNA probes since they are double-stranded and require denaturation. Primers tailed with specific RNA polymerase promoter sequences allow these sequences to be used as templates for transcribing cRNA probes, following an unlabelled PCR reaction (Sitzmann and LeMotte, 1993; Wu *et al.* 1995).

In situ PCR is a technique that has stimulated much controversy and interest (Komminoth and Long, 1993; O'Leary *et al.* 1996). Its aim is to amplify mRNA signals to make visible results that are weak or undetectable by conventional *in situ* hybridization. One approach uses unlabelled PCR reactions in tissue sections, followed by detection of the amplified product by *in situ* hybrid-ization with a labelled probe. Some investigators use riboprobes for the de-tection step, allowing comparisons of native mRNA signals with the amplified results following PCR (Mee *et al.* 1996). Use of a sense riboprobe allows only the amplified product to be detected (Mee *et al.* 1996), since the native mRNA will be the same orientation as the sense probe, whereas the PCR product contains a mixture of sense and antisense sequences.

General procedure for *in situ* hybridization using cRNA probes

The main steps in the procedure will be discussed in sequence. Detailed protocols are provided in the Appendix.

Generation of cRNA probes

RNA probes are obtained by inserting a specific cDNA sequence into an appropriate transcription vector, containing an RNA polymerase promoter (Fig. 4.1). Vectors of this type include the plasmids pSP64 and pSP65, the Gemini vectors, and Bluescript. The last two possess two different promoters

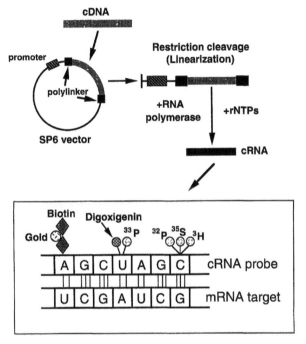

Fig. 4.1. Diagrammatic representation of riboprobe construction.

located on either side of the multiple cloning site. The plasmids pSP64 and pSP65 differ in the orientation of the multiple cloning site in relation to the SP6 promoter. Transcription of 'sense' (control, mRNA sequence) and 'anti-sense' (cRNA sequence) strands can thus be obtained, either by inserting the specific cDNAs into two separate plasmids (pSP64 and pSP65) or into those containing two different promotes, so that the cDNA insert can be transcribed in either direction. The circular plasmid is first linearized by restriction endonuclease digestion within the polylinker, before *in vitro* transcription in order to produce riboprobes of the appropriate length; linearization must be complete to avoid transcription of any contaminating vector sequences. Under appropriate conditions the polymerase will incorporate free ribonucleotides into single-stranded cRNA transcripts of the DNA insert (Fig. 4.1).

Probe labelling

Labelling is carried out using isotopes, detectable autoradiographically, or non-isotopic substances, detectable by immunocytochemical methods. Either type of label is incorporated into the cRNA probe during *in vitro* transcription from the linearized template by use of labelled nucleotides (usually CTP or UTP) in the transcription buffer (see protocol in Appendix). For more information, see Chapters 1–3.

The most commonly used isotopes are β-particle emitters such as ^{32}P, ^{35}S, ^{3}H, or ^{33}P, the latter of which was introduced relatively recently for labelling of nucleotide sequences. Safety is an important consideration in the choice of label, and ^{32}P emits high energy β-particles which have high penetration and may be hazardous. High energy β-particles have wider scatter from the labelled hybrid/cell, so that although results can be obtained quickly, the resolution of the signal may be poor. The other three isotopes emit lower energy particles so can provide better resolution and are less hazardous, but require longer autoradiographic exposures to detect labelled hybrids. Sulfur-35 (^{35}S) can cause problems as a result of non-specific disulfide bonding with the tissue, and ^{3}H requires very long exposures (weeks or months), although it provides high (even subcellular) resolution. Some workers believe that ^{33}P provides advantages over the other isotopes (Evans and Read 1992), since this isotope provides good resolution in short exposure times and without excessive background labelling (McLaughlin and Margolskee 1993), but its high cost may preclude its use.

Non-isotopic labels include digoxigenin, biotin, and FITC, detected immunocytochemically using a variety of techniques, which often provide more flexibility than autoradiography. The FISH technique uses direct detection of probes labelled with fluorescent markers (Ballard and Ward 1993). Non-isotopic labels offer the advantages of safety, speed of detection, high resolution, and longer shelf-life of labelled probes (isotopic probes are only optimal within their half-life range). It has been shown that non-isotopic and isotopic probes can give similar results (Pohle *et al.* 1996) and our experience confirms this finding. Isotopic probes may provide greater sensitivity than non-isotopic probes, but non-isotopic probes give better resolution of the signal at the cellular level.

Tissue preparation

Tissue must be fixed before *in situ* hybridization is carried out, in order to retain nucleic acids in the tissue, preserve the tissue structure, and optimize probe penetration. For further comments on fixatives see Chapter 1. Fixation can be achieved by perfusion or immersion of tissue, or after unfixed frozen tissue has been sectioned. The method of fixation depends on the source of the tissue—perfusion is usually optimal and can be carried out on most small animals, but immersion fixation may be the only available procedure for tissue samples taken from human patients or autopsies, or from larger animals. Frozen sections have been widely used, since the accepted wisdom is that preservation of mRNA is optimal if tissue is frozen rapidly following fixation. However, paraffin-embedded archival tissue can be used successfully when there is likely to be a high copy number of the target sequence (Poulsom *et al.* 1993; Hanby *et al.* 1996). Although some loss of mRNA will occur during paraffin processing, this may be balanced by improved morphology of the tissue and clearer resolution of the final result (Chinery *et al.* 1992). An

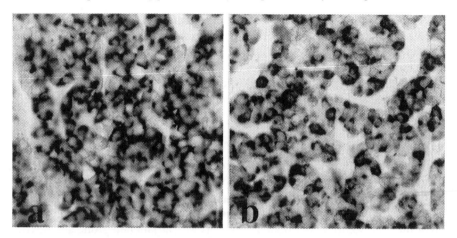

Fig. 4.2. Sections of rat pituitary hybridized with a digoxigenin-labelled prolactin cRNA probe; (a) frozen section (10 μm) and (b) paraffin section (5 μm). Note the improvement in resolution and cellular morphology in the paraffin section, although there is some reduction in staining owing to loss of mRNA during paraffin processing.

example of the difference between results obtained using frozen and paraffin sections is shown in Fig. 4.2.

Prehybridization treatments

Probe penetration is dependent upon the type and extent of fixation, the tissue used, the section thickness, and the length of the probe. Empirical tests with each tissue will be required in order to obtain the optimum conditions. Permeabilization is usually necessary and may be carried out by digestion with proteases such as proteinase K, pronase, or pepsin, or exposure to dilute acids or detergents. Excessive deproteinization may, however, result in loss of tissue structure and diffusion of target RNA. Following protease treatment, it is essential to arrest digestion and this is carried out by immersion in a glycine solution, followed by a brief fixation step in 4% paraformaldehyde. The tissue may then be treated in order to prevent background signals, which may arise through the formation of imperfect duplexes with non-homologous nucleic acids, electrostatic interactions between charged groups, physical entrapment in the three-dimensional lattice of the tissue section, or artefacts of the detection system. Non-specific signal can be reduced by post-hybridization enzyme treatments and stringency washes (see below). Electrostatic interactions between basic proteins in the tissue and the probe itself can sometimes be reduced by treatment with 0.25% acetic anhydride, which blocks basic groups (Tecott *et al.* 1987) and this treatment may be particularly beneficial when using longer probes or probes at higher concentrations. Some investigators also acetylate slides and coverslips to minimize non-specific adherence of probes to glass.

A pre-hybridization solution is sometimes incubated with the sections immediately before application of the hybridization mixture, which is designed to decrease background labelling. This includes components intended to saturate sites in the tissue section that might otherwise bind to nucleic acid non-specifically. These can include ficoll, bovine serum albumin, polyvinyl pyrrolidone, sodium pyrophosphate, and ethylenediamine tetra-acetic acid (EDTA).

Hybridization

Variables that affect the hybridization of the probe to its target include probe length and concentration, stringency of hybridization conditions, stability of hybrids, kinetics of hybridization, and preservation of tissue structure. Hybridization buffer mixtures usually include all the components of the pre-hybridization solution mentioned above, as well as labelled probe and dextran sulfate. Dextran sulfate can greatly amplify hybridization signals and increase the rate of hybridization approximately 10-fold, because nucleic acids are excluded from the volume of the solution occupied by the polymer, thus increasing the effective probe concentration (Wahl *et al.* 1979).

Probe concentration

The optimal concentration may need to be evaluated for each probe, but the criterion should be the concentration that gives the greatest signal-to-noise ratio. Since background noise is linearly related to probe concentration, it is best to use the lowest concentration required to saturate the target mRNA. In our experience, a useful concentration for many probes is 0.5 ng/μl for isotopically labelled probes or 2.5 ng/μl for non-isotopic labels. Excessive probe concentration will give rise to problems with background labelling, but to some extent this can be ameliorated by the use of acetic anhydride before application of the probe. The working concentration of non-isotopic probes can be titrated in a similar way to that in which antibody dilutions are determined for immunocytochemistry.

Probe length

The best length of cRNA probes is thought to be between 50 and 300 nucleotides, but this is dependent upon the tissue concerned. In some cases, probes as long as 1–2 kilobases have been used successfully by us and by others (Wilkinson 1992). Shorter probes can usually penetrate tissues adequately using standard fixation and permeabilization methods, but they form less stable hybrids and may produce higher levels of background as a result of non-specific binding. If necessary, some workers advocate mild hydrolysis of longer probes prior to hybridization (see Appendix), but our experience suggests that this can lead to artefacts. Alternatively, probe design with shorter DNA fragments cloned in an appropriate vector system can ensure that probes of optimal length are generated.

Stringency

Stringency increases with temperature and formamide concentration, and is inversely related to salt concentration, and is important when performing *in situ* hybridization and carrying out post-hybridization washes. Duplexes with high sequence homology withstand high stringency conditions better than duplexes with low homology; therefore, increased stringency can be used to loosen non-specific bonds between probe and nucleic acids. The melting temperatures (T_m) of probes and hybrids depend upon nucleotide composition and their length. Since hybridization is generally performed at relatively low temperatures in order to preserve tissue structure and ensure that the probe remains intact, non-specific interactions may occur, and post-hybridization washing of increased stringency is necessary to dissociate non-homologous hybrids. The choice of stringency conditions of hybridization itself must be determined by the use of a range of temperatures and salt concentrations, in order to select the optimum. It is important to choose a temperature at which the tissue structure preservation is also optimized. In our experience, temperatures up to 55°C can be used for washes without harming tissue.

Stability of hybrids

Factors that enhance hybrid stability include high ionic strength, high salt concentration, and a high percentage of GC base pairs. By contrast, formamide disrupts hydrogen bonds and hence has a destabilizing effect, but it is included in most hybridization reactions as a means of preventing the association of non-homologous strands at the relatively low temperatures required to maintain tissue structure. The increased stability of RNA–RNA bonds, in comparison with DNA–RNA bonds, means that *in situ* hybridization with cRNA probes can be carried out at higher hybridization temperatures (by about 10–15°C) than hybridization with other probes of comparable length and GC content (Cox *et al.* 1984).

Post-hybridization treatments

Post-hybridization washes of increasing stringency ensure dissociation of non-homologous hybrids. The high levels of non-specific binding incurred by using RNA probes can be removed effectively by post-hybridization treatment with RNase. Under appropriate conditions, RNase selectively removes non-base paired RNA from tissue sections, reducing background with little loss of specific signal. The acceptable level of background depends upon the expected length of exposure and the intensity of the specific signal; if a long exposure is anticipated and high resolution is required, more extensive washing may be necessary. The protocol in the Appendix gives standard stringency conditions, but the washes can be adapted by introducing washes of lower salt concentrations and/or increasing temperature, to remove more of the non-specifically bound, imperfect hybrids. A series of stringency washes typically includes buffers of decreasing salt concentration and sometimes formamide is included. As in the protocol provided here, detergents such as sodium dodecyl sulfate (SDS) can be added to the washing buffer to speed up the dissociation of non-specific binding.

Detection systems

Isotopic probes (autoradiography)

Isotopically labelled hybrids are visualized using autoradiographic procedures. Depending upon the degree of sensitivity and resolution required, slides can be apposed directly to X-ray film (specially designed for the detection of β-particles, e.g. Amersham β-Max), or dipped into molten nuclear emulsion (e.g. Ilford K5). In either case, the slides are exposed to the film or emulsion in darkness and a darkroom is required. The first method is rapid, with exposure times ranging from several hours to 2–3 days, and this can provide a quick assessment of probe binding and rough distribution in the tissue, but the sensitivity and resolution are low and no microscopic detail can be seen. Alternatively, slides can be dipped in liquid nuclear track emulsion, to localize mRNA at the cellular level, and the autoradiographic signal can then be viewed microscopically. The length of exposure depends upon the level of mRNA present and the isotope used for probe labelling. Exposure times range from 3–15 days for ^{32}P, ^{33}P, or ^{35}S, to 6–18 weeks for ^{3}H. The optimal exposure time should be determined for each experiment, balancing the increase in signal as time progresses with the corresponding increase in background noise. The signal-to-noise ratio requires optimization and the autoradiographs should be developed when the specific signal reaches the maximum level (after which point the background will continue to increase without further increase in specific signal). Duplicate test slides should be included so that exposure times for the particular probe and tissue in question can be determined. Counterstaining of the tissue section beneath the emulsion layer, with stains such as haematoxylin or Giemsa, reveals the tissue structure and allows precise localization of the bound probe.

Non-isotopic probes

Visualization of non-isotopically labelled hybrids may be achieved by using various immunocytochemical methods, providing good cellular resolution. A wide variety of immunocytochemical systems is available. For the most popular non-isotopic label, digoxigenin (Black *et al.* 1993; Steel *et al.* 1994; Terenghi and Polak 1994), antidigoxigenin antibodies are available, labelled directly with fluorochromes such as FITC, or with colloidal gold (Boehringer Mannheim). Unlabelled antidigoxen monoclonal antibody (Sigma) can detect digoxigenin at high dilutions and allows multilayer immunocytochemical methods to be used. Biotinylated probes can be detected using avidin or streptavidin systems (Block 1993), by virtue of the extremely strong bond formed between biotin and avidin. Development of peroxidase systems can be carried out using conventional immunocytochemical methods such as 3′,3-diaminobenzidine (DAB) or the nickel–DAB–glucose oxidase method (Shu *et al.* 1988). If gold-labelled reagents are used, enhancement with silver ions can provide a light microscope-visible product with high sensitivity (Springall *et al.* 1984), or the gold label can be applied to electron microscopy (Lackie *et al.* 1989). Selection of reaction products of different colours can allow co-localization studies to be carried out, or combination with other techniques such as immunocytochemistry. In addition, it is possible to detect multiple mRNAs using a combination of isotopically and non-isotopically labelled probes (Miller *et al.* 1993).

Determination of specificity

Before using a probe for *in situ* hybridization, its size and integrity should be confirmed by electrophoresis, using polyacrylamide gel electrophoresis, and its specificity established by Northern blotting. When applying the probe to tissue sections, it is essential to verify the specificity of hybridization signals by including appropriate controls (Tecott *et al.* 1987; see Chapter 1). A variety of controls may be used: pre-treatment of the tissue with RNase, use of sense probes (with an identical sequence to the target mRNA), heterologous (unrelated) probes, use of multiple probes for a single target, and inhibition of specific binding of labelled probe by competition with unlabelled probe. Inclusion of positive control tissue, or another probe known to provide good results on the tissue concerned, can serve as a method control, and comparison with detection of antigen by means of immunocytochemistry can also provide information about the authenticity of the results. If all the negative controls result in an absence of signal, it is possible to interpret a detectable signal in test sections as genuine and specific.

Quantification

In situ hybridization results can be quantified using computer-assisted image analysis systems (Baskin and Stahl 1993; Rossmanith *et al.* 1996). For more details, see also Chapters 5 and 6. Many factors must be considered if quantitative measurements are required, in order to ensure standardization of the method and reproducibility of the results. Section thickness, probe concentration and label incorporation, hybridization temperature and duration, exposure time and development conditions, and thickness and uniformity of emulsion coating, can affect the intensity of the resulting signal. On the whole, autoradiography is a quantitative process and may be more adaptable to quantification than non-isotopic labels. Autoradiographic results can be quantified by grain counting (Mee *et al.* 1996; Rossmanith *et al.* 1996). For non-isotopic probes, standardization of immunocytochemical detection methods is required, for example by ensuring the development of all slides simultaneously. Standard curves are essential for the calibration of quantitative detection systems, and providing all variables are carefully controlled, data from hybridization results may provide a useful assessment of comparative gene expression or even absolute levels of nucleic acid in a tissue section.

Combined *in situ* hybridization and immunocytochemistry

In situ hybridization can be combined with immunocytochemistry to allow comparison of gene transcription (mRNA) with translation into stored protein. The detection of mRNAs and translated proteins can yield useful information regarding the dynamic status of tissues and cells; for example, a positive *in situ* hybridization signal in the absence of immunoreactivity for the same gene product could suggest high turnover of synthesis and secretion, with no storage of the protein in the cell. Alternatively, immunoreactivity without detectable mRNA could suggest that the antigen is stored in the cell after uptake from the circulation, or that the cell is not actively transcribing the specific gene but still contains intracellular stores of the antigen. These methods can be combined by carrying out each technique on separate sections, using serial sections from the same tissue, with subsequent comparison for co-localization (Steel *et al*. 1988), or by simultaneous detection on the same section (Höfler *et al*. 1987; Steel *et al*. 1990). The latter method has the advantage of better resolution of mRNA and protein but requires optimization of each protocol for the detection of each target molecule.

Double *in situ* hybridization

Recently, the use of two or more cRNA probes for simultaneous *in situ* hybridization on the same section has become more widely used. This approach has been used for detection of multiple mRNAs in certain cell types, mainly in hypothalamic neurones (Grossman *et al*. 1994; Merchant and Miller 1994; Aguilera *et al*. 1995; Rossmanith *et al* 1996). Each probe is labelled with a different reporter and usually an isotopic and non-isotopic probe are combined to allow completely clear, separate detection of the individual signals.

Specific illustrative examples

The following examples have been chosen to illustrate the use of *in situ* hybridization with cRNA probes, (a) to assess endocrine cell activity and (b) when other suitable methods cannot be utilized, in this case for the detection of peptide receptors.

Assessment of endocrine cell activity

The production of hormones by cells of the anterior pituitary gland is under hormonal control, by hypothalamic releasing factors and by feedback of hormones secreted by peripheral endocrine glands. Regulation of pituitary hormone gene expression can take place at the cellular level and therefore *in situ* hybridization is a valuable technique for investigating changes in intracellular mRNA content and the effect of alterations in the endocrine environment. Thyroid stimulating hormone (TSH) gene expression is regulated by thyroid hormones and so changes in thyroid function are expected to modulate TSH expression. A study was carried out to investigate the effect of thyroidectomy on TSH mRNA levels in rat pituitaries (Steel *et al.* 1990). Sections of normal and thyroidectomized rat pituitary were hybridized with a TSH cRNA probe labelled with [32]P. A marked increase in TSH mRNA labelling signal was seen in the thyroidectomized rats compared with controls, with more positive cells present per section and a greater intensity of labelling per cell (Fig. 4.3). There was considerable variation in labelling intensity

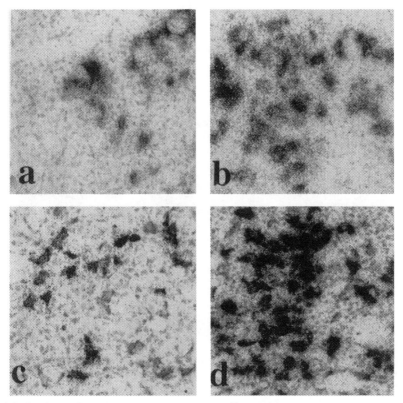

Fig. 4.3. Sections of rat pituitary hybridized with a ^{32}P-labelled rat β-TSG cRNA probe; (a) control and (b) hypothyroid pituitaries provide a comparison of β-TSH mRNA levels, but cellular resolution is poor. Sections from (c) control and (d) hypothyroid pituitaries hybridized first with the probe and subsequently immunostained for rat β-TSH demonstrates the stored protein and mRNA in the same cells. All sections were counterstained with haematoxylin.

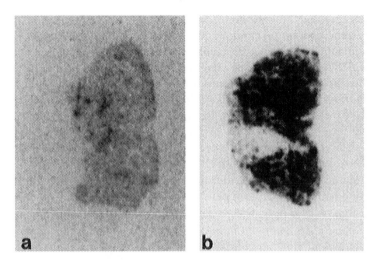

Fig. 4.4. Images from a film autoradiograph of rat pituitary sections hybridized with a ^{35}S-labelled rat β-TSH cRNA probe; (a) control and (b) hypothyroid rat, showing a 20-fold increase in overall labelling intensity.

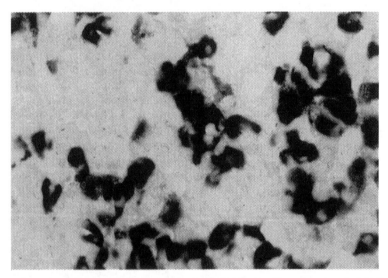

Fig. 4.5. A section of hypothyroid rat pituitaries hybridized with a digoxigenin-labelled rat β-TSH cRNA probe. The resolution of this detection system is greater than with isotopic probes (as in Fig. 4.3).

between individual TSH cells in normal rats, so in order to visualize all the TSH cells in the section more effectively, immunocytochemistry for TSH was carried out following hybridization but before dipping the slides in emulsion. In normal and thyroidectomized rats, TSH mRNA was co-localized with TSH

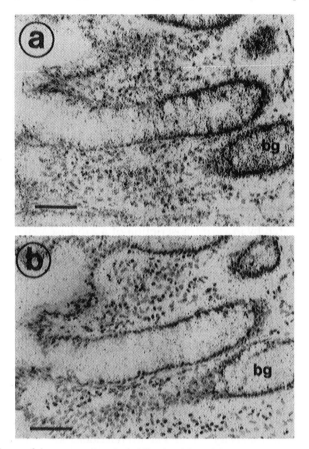

Fig. 4.6. Sections of human colon hybridized with a NPY Y1 receptor cRNA probe; (a) signal is localized autoradiographically to the basal glands (labelled 'bg') and colonic mucosa after 4 days exposure, and (b) a negative control was provided by incubating a duplicate section with a sense probe. The preparations were lightly counterstained with haematoxylin.

immunoreactivity, as expected, and it became clear that some TSH cells in normal rats contained very little TSH mRNA signal, whereas in thyroid-ectomized rats all the TSH immunoreactive cells were intensely labelled for TSH mRNA (Fig. 4.3). This indicated that TSH gene expression is up-regulated at the cellular level after thyroidectomy. In order to quantify the increase, hybridized sections of normal and thyroidectomized rat pituitaries were apposed to X-ray film and images were obtained (Fig. 4.4). The grey level of the images was measured by computer-assisted image analysis with reference to a series of standards, providing a density measurement for the labelling. In sections from thyroidectomized rats, the images had a mean grey level 20-fold higher than in normal rats. Finally, non-isotopic, digoxigenin-labelled probes were used to obtain higher resolution of the TSH mRNA. The bound hybrids were detected using an alkaline phosphatase-conjugated anti-digoxigenin antibody and the enzyme label was visualized with nitroblue tetrazolium chloride and 5-bromo-4-chloro-3-inndoyl phosphate, giving a blue-black product (Fig. 4.5).

Detection of peptide receptor mRNA

The localization of receptors for the neurotransmitter known as neuropeptide tyrosine (NPY) in sections of human tissues has not been achieved using *in vitro* receptor autoradiography, possibly because of a differential species-specific peptide conformation. We were able to localize the expression of the NPY Y1 receptor subtype in human tissue by adopting the technique of *in situ* hybridization (Wharton *et al.* 1993) using ^{35}S-labelled NPY receptor ribo-probes, generated by *in vitro* transcription of a 276 base pair fragment of the human cDNA. The distribution of NPY receptor Y1 mRNA in colon, kidney, adrenal gland, heart, and placenta was investigated and the results indicated a tissue-specific regulation of expression (Fig. 4.6).

References

Aguilera, G., Young, W.S., Kiss, A., and Bathia, A. (1995). Direct regulation of hypothalamic corticotropin-releasing-hormone neurons by angiotensin II. *Neuro-endocrinology*, **61**, 437–44.

Ballard, S.G. and Ward, D.C. (1993). Fluorescence *in situ* hybridization using digital imaging microscopy. *J. Histochem. Cytochem.*, **41**, 1755–60.

Baskin, D.G. and Stahl, W.L. (1993). Fundamentals of quantitative autoradiography by computer densitometry for *in situ* hybridization, with emphasis on ^{33}P. *J. Hitochem. Cytochem.*, **41**, 1767–76.

Black, M., Carey, F.A., Farquharson, M.A., Murray, G.D., and McNicol, A.M. (1993). Expression of the pro-opiomelanocortin gene in lung neuroendocrine tumours: *in situ* hybridization and immunocytochemical studies. *J. Pathol.*, **169**, 329–34.

Bloch, B. (1993). Biotinylated probes for *in situ* hybridization histochemistry: use for mRNA detection. *J. Histochem. Cytochem.*, **41**, 1751–4.

Chinery, R., Poulsom, R., Rogers, L., Jeffery, R.E., Longcroft, J.M., Hanby, A.M., and Wright, N.A. (1992). Localization of intestinal trefoil-factor mRNA in rat stomach and intestine by hybridization *in situ*. *Biochem. J.*, **285**, 5–8.

Cox, K.H., DeLeon, D.V., Angerer, L.M., and Angerer, R.C. (1984). Detection of mRNAs in sea urchin embryos by *in situ* hybridization using asymmetric RNA probes. *Dev. Biol.*, **101**, 485–502.

Denny, P., Hamid, Q., Krause, J.M., Polak, J.M., and Legon, S. (1988). Oligo-riboprobes: tools for *in situ* hybridization. *Histochemistry*, **89**, 481–3.

Evans, M.R. and Read, C.A. (1992). ^{32}P, ^{33}P and ^{35}S: selecting a label for nucleic acid analysis. *Nature*, **358**, 520–1.

Grossman, A.B., Rossmanith, W.G., Kabigting, E.B., Cadd, G., Clifton, D., and Steiner, R.A. (1994). The distribution of hypothalamic nitric oxide synthase mRNA in relation to gonadotrophin-releasing hormone neurons. *J. Endocrinol.*, **140**, R5–R8.

Hanby, A.M., Chinery, R., Poulsom, R., Playford, R.J., and Pignatelli, M. (1996). Downregulation of E-cadherin in the reparative epithelium of the human gastrointestinal tract. *Am. J. Pathol.*, **148**, 723–9.

Höfler, H., Pütz, B., Ruhri, C., Wirnsberger, G., Klimpfinger, M., and Smolle, J. (1987). Simultaneous localization of calcitonin mRNA and peptide in a medullary thyroid carcinoma. *Virch. Archiv B*, **54**, 144–51.

Komminoth, P. and Long, A.A. (1993). *In-situ* polymerase chain reaction. An overview of methods, applications and limitations of a new molecular technique. *Virch. Arch. V, Cell. Pathol. Incl. Mol. Pathol.*, **64**, 67–73.

Lackie, P.M., Hennessy, R.J., Hacker, G.W., and Polak, J.M. (1989). Investigation of immunogold–silver staining by electron microscopy. *Histochemistry*, **83**, 545–50.

McLaughlin, S.K. and Margolskee, R.F. (1993). P-33 is preferable to S-35 for labelling probes used in *in situ* hybridization. *Biotechniques*, **15**, 506–11.

Mee, A.P., Hoyland, J.A., Braidman, I.P., Freemont, A.J., Davies, M., and Mawer, E.B. (1996). Demonstration of vitamin D receptor transcripts in actively resorbing osteclasts in bone sections. *Bone*, **18**, 295–9.

Merchant, K.M. and Miller, M.A. (1994). Coexpression of neurotensin and c-fos mRNAs in rat neostriatal neurons following acute haloperidol. *Brain Res. Mol. Brain Res.*, **23**, 271–7.

Miller, M.A., Kolb, P.E., and Raskind, M.A. (1993). A method for simultaneous detection of multiple mRNAs using digoxigenin and radioisotopic cRNA probes. *J. Histochem. Cytochem.*, **41**, 1741–50.

O'Leary, J.J., Chetty, R., Graham, A.K., and McGee, J.O'D. (1996). *In situ* PCR: pathologist's dream or nightmare? *J. Pathol*, **178**, 11–20.

Pohle, T., Shahin, M., Gillessen, A., Schuppan, D., Herbst, H., and Domschke, W. (1996). Expression of type I and IV collagen mRNAs in healing gastric ulcers—a comparative analysis using isotopic and non-radioactive *in situ* hybridization. *Histochem. Cell Biol.*, **106**, 413–18.

Poulsom, R., Hanby, A.M., Pignatelli, M., Jeffery, R.E., Longcroft, J.M., Rogers, L., and Stamp, G.W. (1993). Expression of gelatinase A and TIMP-2 mRNAs in desmoplastic fibroblasts in both mammary carcinomas and basal cell carcinomas of the skin. *J. Clin. Pathol.*, **46**, 429–36.

Rossmanith, W.G., Marks, D.L., Clifton, D. K., and Steiner, R.A. (1996). Induction of galanin mRNA in GnRH neurons by estradiol and its facilitation by progesterone. *J. Neuroendocrinol.*, **8**, 185–91.

Shu, S., Ju, G., and Fan, L. (1988). The glucose oxidase–DAB–nickel method in peroxidase histochemistry of the nervous system. *Neurosci. Lett.*, **85**, 169–71.

Sitzmann, J.H. and LeMotte, P.K. (1993). Rapid and efficient generation of PCR-derived riboprobe templates for *in situ* hybridization histochemistry. *J. Histochem Cytochem.*, **41**, 773–6.

Springall, D.R., Hacker, G.W., Grimelius, G.W., and Polak, J.M. (1984). The potential of the immunogold–silver staining method for paraffin sections. *Histochemistry*, **81**, 603–8.

Steel, J.H., Hamid, Q., Van Noorden, S., Jones, P., Denny, P., Burrin, J., Legon, S., Bloom, S.R., and Polak, J.M. (1988). Combined use of *in situ* hybridization and immunocytochemistry for the investigation of prolactin gene expression in immature, pubertal, pregnant, lactating and ovariectomized rats. *Histochemistry*, **89**, 75–80.

Steel, J.H., O'Halloran, D.J., Jones, P.M., Van Noorden, S., Chin, W.W., Bloom, S.R., and Polak, J.M. (1990). Combined use of immunocytochemistry and *in situ* hybridization to study β-thyroid-stimulating hormone gene expression in pituitaries of hypothyroid rats. *Mol. Cell. Probes*, **4**, 385–96.

Steel, J.H., Martínez, A., Springall, D.R., Treston, A.M., Cuttitta, F., and Polak, J.M. (1994). Peptidylglycine α-amidating monooxygenase immunoreactivity and messenger RNA in human pituitary and increased expression in pituitary tumours. *Cell. Tissue Res.*, **276**, 197–207.

Tecott, L.H., Eberwine, J.H., Barchas, J.D., and Valentino, K.L. (1987). Methodological consideration in the utilization of *in situ* hybridization. In: *In situ* hybridization: applications to neurobiology, (eds K.L. Valentino, J.H. Eberwine, and J.D. Barchas). Oxford University Press, New York.

Terenghi, G. and Polak, J.M. (1994). Detecting mRNA in tissue sections with digoxigenin-labeled probes. *Meth. Mol. Biol.*, **28**, 193–9.

Wahl, G.M., Stern, M., and Stark, G.R. (1979). Efficient transfer of large DNA fragments from agarose gels to diazobenzylomethyl-paper and rapid hybridization by using dextran sulfate. *Proc. Natl. Acad. Sci. USA*, **76**, 3683–7.

Wetmur, J.G., Ruyechan, W.T., and Douthart, R.J. (1981). Denaturation and renaturation of *Penicillium chrysogenum* mycophage double-stranded ribonucleic acid in tetraalkylammonium salt solutions. *Biochemistry*, **20**, 2999–3002.

Wharton, J., Gordon, L., Byrne, J., Moore, K., Sullivan, M.H.F., Elder, M.G., Moscoso, G., Taylor, K.M., Shine, J., and Polak, J.M. (1993). Expression of the human neuropeptide tyrosine (NPY)—Y1 receptor. *Proc. Nat. Acad. Sci. USA*, **90**, 687–91.

Wilkinson, D.G. (1992). *In situ hybridization. A practical approach*. Oxford University Press, Oxford.

Wu, H., Wang, D., and Malarkey, W.B. (1995). A PCR-derived, non-isotopic labeled prolactin cRNA probe suitable for *in situ* hybridization. *Endocrinol Res.*, **21**, 793–802.

Appendix 4.1. Protocols

Protocol 1. Generation of complementary RNA probe

1. cDNA, cloned in an appropriate vector, is purified by phenol–chloroform extraction or by using one of the DNA preparation kits that are commercially available).

2. The vector is linearized at a point in the cloning site of the polylinker, using an appropriate restriction enzyme, to allow for transcription of probe of the required orientation (antisense or sense) and is finally purified and resuspended in Tris–EDTA buffer (Tris, 10 mM; EDTA, 0.1 mM; pH8) to a concentration of 1 μg/μl.

3. The following components are added to a sterile RNase-free microcentrifuge tube at room temperature.

- 5 × transcription buffer*   2 µl
- 400 mM dithiothreitol (DTT)   1 µl
- Linearized plasmid template DNA (1 µg/µl)   1 µl
- Isotopically labelled nucleotide, e.g. ^{32}P-CTP (20 µCi/µl)   5 µl

  (*Non-isotopically labelled nucleotide, eg.*   1 µl
  digoxigenin-UTP, 10 mM
  isotopically labelled tracer, eg. ^{32}P-CTP   1 µl)

- RNA polymerase (20 U/µl)   1 µl

Add water to a final volume of 10 µl, mix gently and incubate at 37°C for 1 h.

4. Transcription is terminated by removing the template: add 1 µl DNase (RNase-free, 1 mg/ml) and incubate at 37°C for 10 mins.

5. The total volume is made up to 200 µl with RNase-free water and unincorporated nucleotides and enzymes are removed by phenol–chloroform extraction (1:1, saturated with Tris) and chloroform–isoamyl alcohol (24:1) extractions.

6. The incorporation of the labelled nucleotide is calculated from the ratio of dpm counted on two filters, each spotted with 1 µl of the water-diluted reaction mixture in step 5 before the phenol–chloroform extraction step. One filter (A) is kept dry and the other (B) is washed to remove unincorporated labelled nucleotides, as follows: 0.5M Na_2HPO_4, 6 × 5 mins; distilled water, 2 × 1 min; and absolute alcohol, 2 × 1 min. The washed filter is air dried and both filters are counted in a scintillation counter. % incorporation = (cpm filter B/cpm filter A) × 100. 100% incorporation provides 165 ng of probe, so that the total yield of probe can be calculated.

7. After the extraction steps, the aqueous supernatant containing the RNA probe is precipitated by adding:

- ammonium acetate   final concentration of 2.5 M
- ethanol   2.5 volumes (ice-cold)
- glycogen (20 mg/ml)   2 µl

Store at −20°C for 2 h and spin for 15 min, wash pellet in 70% alcohol and spin again for 5 min, dry pellet and resuspend in sterile water or Tris–EDTA at a concentration of 5 ng/µl.

* Transcription buffer: 200 mM Tris–HCl (pH 7.5), 40 mM $MgCl_2$, 10 mM spermidine trihydrochloride, 50 mM DTT, 0.5 mg/ml bovine serum albumin (BSA), 500 U/ml ribonuclease inhibitor, 2.5 mM of each unlabelled nucleotide, eg. ATP, GTP, and UTP (or ATP, GTP, and CTP).

Protocol 2.   Probe hydrolysis

1. Probe is dissolved in sterile water as above, and the following are added:
    - water   160 μl
    - $NaHCO_3$ (0.4 M)   20 μl
    - Na_2CO_3 (0.6 M)   20 μl

    Mix well and incubate at 60°C for the appropriate time interval (see step 2).

2. The incubation time for hydrolysis is calculated as follows:

$$t = \frac{L_0 - L_f}{kL_0L_f}$$

where t = time (min); L_0 = original length of probe (kb); L_f = required final length of probe (kb); k = rate constant for hydrolysis (0.11 kb/min).

3. Hydrolysis is terminated by adding sodium acetate to a final concentration of 0.1 M and glacial acetic acid to 0.5% v/v.

4. Probe is precipitated (as in Protocol 1) and resuspended to a final concentration of 5 ng/μl for an isotopically labelled probe or 25 ng/μl for a non-isotopically labelled probe, after estimating probe recovery.

Protocol 3.   Tissue preparation

1. For animal tissues, the optimum method of fixation is perfusion, followed by post-fixation for 2–4 h. For immersion fixation, the tissue is dissected and placed in 4% paraformaldehyde in 0.1 M phosphate buffered saline (PBS, pH 7.2) for 6 h at 4°C. The ratio of tissue to fixative should be greater than 1:10.

2. The tissue is then rinsed repeatedly in PBS containing 15% sucrose and 0.1% sodium azide, for at least 24 h.

3. Cryostat blocks are prepared by orienting the tissue on to cork circles, surrounding it with mounting medium such as TissueTek OCT medium, and rapidly freezing it in melting isopentane/liquid nitrogen. Tissue blocks re then stored at −40 or −70°C.

4. Tissue is sectioned to a thickness of 10 μm in a cryostat at −25°C, sections are thaw-mounted on to Vectabond-treated RNase-free glass slides and are dried thoroughly before processing for ISH. Dried sections can be stored at −70°C with desiccant.

Protocol 4. Tissue pre-treatment

1. Cryostat sections are rehydrated and permeabilized by immersion in detergent: 0.2% Triton X-100 in PBS for 15 min.

2. Rinse twice in PBS for 3 mins each.

3. Protease digestion is carried out by incubating sections with proteinase K ($1\mu g/ml$) in 0.1 M Tris–0.05 M EDTA (pH 8) at 37 °C for up to 20 min (the appropriate incubation time for each tissue should be determined in a preliminary experiment to make sure that the tissue structure is not destroyed. Some tissues, eg. pancrease, do not require any protease treatment).

4. Inactivate the enzyme by immersing slides in 0.1M glycine in PBS for 5 min at room temperature.

5. Briefly (3 min) post-fix with 4% paraformaldehyde in PBS to prevent possible diffusion of target nucleic acid.

6. Rinse briefly in PBS twice.

7. Immerse slides in 0.25% acetic anhydride in 0.1M triethanolamine (pH8) for 10 min with agitation (acetylates tissue and prevents non-specific binding of probe).

8. Rinse slides briefly in distilled water. Air dry sections at 37 °C for about 10 min. An RNase-treated control section may be included to confirm the nature of the material to which probe is bound. Before protease treatment, a section is incubated with a solution of RNase (100 μg/ml, DNase-free) for 30 min at 37 °C. After this, the slide is processed as normal, but care must be taken to avoid contaminating the test sections with RNase.

Protocol 5. Hybridization

1. The probe is diluted 1:10 in hybridization buffer (see below) to a final concentration of 0.5 ng/μl (isotopic) or 2.5 ng/μl (non-isotopic).

   Hybridization buffer (may be stored, in aliquots, at -20 °C. Do not repeatedly freeze–thaw): 50% deionized formamide; 5 × standard saline citrate (SSC, see below); 10% w/v dextran sulfate (added at 50 °C); 5 × Denhard't solution (see below); 2% w/v sodium dodecyl sulfate (SDS); 100 μg/ml herring sperm DNA (denatured and sheared).

   • Denhardt's solution (100 ×): 10 g Ficoll, 10 g polyvinylpyrrolidone (PVP), 10 g BSA, 500 ml sterile water.

   • Standard saline citrate (20 ×): 175.3 g sodium chloride and 88.2 g sodium citrate, made up to 1 litre with double-distilled water.

2. 10 μl of diluted probe is applied to each section and a siliconized coverslip is placed on top, before incubating slides at the desired temperature in a humid chamber for 12–18 h. The temperature selected may be from 37°C (oligoprobes) up to 60°C, depending upon the T_m for each probe. We normally start at 42°C for riboprobes, and conditions can be modified on the basis of these results.

Protocol 6. Stringency washes

1. The coverslips are gently removed by immersing the slides in 2 ×SSC/0.1% SDS.
2. Wash the slides in 2 × SSC/0.1% SDS for 4 × 5 min at room temperature with gentle shaking.
3. Wash in 0.1 × SSC/0.1% SDS for 2 × 10 min at the temperature used for hybridization.
4. Rinse thoroughly in 2 × SSC to remove all traces of SDS.
5. Incubate sections in RNase (10 μg/μl) in 2 × SSC at 37°C for 15 mins.
6. Rinse briefly in 2 × SSC.
7. If processing for autoradiography, dehydrate in graded alcohols (70, 90, and 100% ethanol) containing 0.3 M ammonium acetate and dry thoroughly at room temperature. Proceed to Protocol 7. If processing slides for immunocytochemical detection, do not dehydrate, but proceed to Protocol 8.

Protocol 7. Autoradiography

Appropriate safe-light filters for use with autoradiographic emulsion/film are given in the manufacturers product specifications. All procedures are carried out in a dark room.

1. Sections may be apposed to autoradiographic film (Amersham β-max Hyperfilm) for the desired time (depending on the isotope). The film is then developed in Kodak D19 developer for 5 min at 20°C, washed in a 0.2% solution of glacial acetic acid, and fixed for 10 min in a 20% solution of photographic fixer. The film is rinsed thoroughly in running tap water followed by a rinse in distilled water prior to drying.
2. Nuclear track emulsion (Amersham LM1, Ilford K5) is melted at 45°C and poured into a glass dipping chamber where it is allowed to settle until air bubbles disperse. The slides are warmed on a hot-plate to the same

temperature, to prevent cooling of the emulsion, and are gently dipped and then dried for 1–2 h at room temperature in a vertical position. When dry, slides are placed in light-tight boxes with desiccant and stored at 4 °C for the required exposure time. Slides are developed in Kodak D19 for 3 min at 20 °C, rinsed in water and fixed for 5–8 min. The slides are washed thoroughly, counterstained with haematoxylin and carefully dehydrated and mounted. Appropriate exposure times are determined by trial and error and by the use of duplicate test slides in every batch.

Protocol 8. Visualization of digoxigenin-labelled probes

1. Slides are rinsed in buffer containing 0.1 M Tris (pH 7.5), 0.1 M NaCl, 2 mM $MgCl_2$ (Buffer 1) for 2 × 3 min.

2. Non-specific antibody binding is blocked by immersion in Buffer 1 containing 3% BSA for 10 min.

3. Alkaline phosphatase-labelled anti-digoxigenin antibody, diluted 1:500 in buffer 1, is applied to sections and incubated for 2 h at room temperature.

4. Sections are washed in Buffer 1 for 3 × 3 min.

5. Sections are placed in Buffer 2 [0.1 M Tris (pH 9.5), 0.1 M NaCl and 0.5 mM $MgCl_2$] prior to incubation in substrate solution.

6. The slides are then incubated in substrate solution [Buffer 2 containing 1 mM levamisole (to block endogenous enzyme), 330 μl nitroblue tetra-zolium solution (NBT: 10 mg/ml) and 33 μl 5-bromo-3-chloro-3-indoyl phos-phate stock solution (BCIP: 25 mg in 1 ml dimethylformamide), NBT and BCIP available from Sigma), for 5–20 min, in darkness. In some cases, longer incubation at 4 °C may give good results. Alternative strategies for visualization of non-isotopic probes are described in Boehringer Mannheim's Application Manual.

5

Quantification of *in situ* hybridization macro-autoradiograms

ANTHONY P. DAVENPORT

Introduction

In situ hybridization uses single-stranded polynucleotide probes to detect endogenous nucleic acids in slide-mounted sections of tissue. Incorporation of a radioactive reporter molecule within these probes permits the precise anatomical localization and quantification of mRNA encoding a range of biologically active molecules, including transmitters, receptors, and enzymes, using autoradiography and image analysis.

Two autoradiographical detection methods can be employed depending on the level of resolution required. Using micro-autoradiography, radioactivity is detected when viewed under the microscope as the pattern of individual silver grains in a thin layer of nuclear emulsion lying above the tissue. This is applied either by dipping the slides into liquid emulsion or by apposition to emulsion-coated coverslips. Radioactivity and, therefore, the amount of probe hybridized can be measured by counting the number of silver grains per cell or unit area lying directly above the specimen and is described in detail in Chapter 6.

A limitation of quantitative micro-autoradiography is that measurement of grain density can be difficult to make with precision because a number of factors may affect the response of the emulsion to radioactivity; although Jonker *et al.* (1997) found that the results obtained by measuring the integrated density of silver grains produced in tissue sections following *in situ* hybridization were directly proportional to the signal measured by Northern blot analysis. These factors include the characteristics of the radiation source, the length of exposure, and the conditions of development (for detailed discussion see Rogers 1979). For example, isotopes such as ^{35}S and ^{32}P, emit β-particles of sufficiently high energy to pass through the emulsion, and, under these conditions, grain densities may vary with emulsion thickness (Young and Kuhar 1986). This problem can be avoided by the use of tritium to label the probes, since this isotope produces particles with a maximum range in emulsion of about 2 μm. Provided the emulsion is 10–15 μm thick all β-particles emitted in the direction of the emulsion should be detected. However, variation in tissue density can result in differential self absorption of the low energy particles emitted by tritium, producing errors in measuring the concentration of radioactivity and, therefore, the amount of probe hybridized in a single cell.

Macro-autoradiography can be used when single cell resolution is not required. In this method, sections of radiolabelled tissue are exposed to nuclear emulsion coated on to film. The main advantage is that factors that alter the response of the emulsion to radioactivity can be controlled for or avoided by co-exposing the radiolabelled sections with a set of calibrated standards that resembles the experimental source. At the end of the exposure period, the film is separated from the slides and, after development, the resulting pattern of optical densities within the autoradiograms can be quantified by comparison with a standard curve generated from the calibrated radioactive scale using computer-assisted densitometry. Radioactivity and, therefore, the amount of probe hybridizing to groups of cells can be measured.

In situ hybridization has a number of advantages compared with other methods of detecting mRNA, such as solution hybridization or Northern blotting, which both require the homogenization of tissue to extract the mRNA. Because the morphology of the tissue section is retained, *in situ* hybridization can be very sensitive. One assay has been calculated to be able to detect less than five copies per cell of atrial natriuretic factor mRNA in the heart (Nunez *et al.* 1989). This can be important where tissue levels may be low, such as mRNA encoding receptors (Molenaar *et al.* 1993; Davenport *et al.* 1994, 1995). The technique is particularly valuable in complex structures such as the brain, where the expression of many genes coding for enzymes, neurotransmitters, or receptors may be localized to discrete nuclei that represent only a small fraction of the total cells (see, for example, Tracer and Loh 1993 Baubet *et al.* 1994; Eastwood *et al.* 1994). Since a single brain section may contain 60–70 anatomically defined regions, different areas can be examined without pre-selection of the tissue. This can be important where lesions are performed resulting in an increase in mRNA in one region which is balanced by a loss in another (Tracer and Loh 1993). Techniques based on homogenization of large samples of brain may not detect such a change. *In situ* hybridization can be carried out with sections 10 μm thick, or less, which is important when the supply of tissue is limited, particularly with human samples obtained during surgery or from biopsies. In addition, consecutive sections can be employed to compare multiple probes directed to the same mRNA, or probes directed to other mRNAs coding for different proteins. *In situ* hybridization can be combined with other neurochemical methods, particularly ligand binding (Radja *et al.* 1993) and immunocytochemistry (Eastwood *et al.* 1994), where the expression of a protein in the CNS (central nervous system) can be correlated with presence of its mRNA.

The aim of this chapter is to describe how macro-autoradiography can be used to localize and quantify cells containing a specific nucleic acid sequence in sections of tissue. Selection of the most appropriate protocols for quantification of mRNA together with possible errors and strategies for avoiding them are discussed. Chapter 1–4 should be consulted for details of the principles of *in situ* hybridization and the design of probes, as well as reviews or original papers by Penschow *et al.* (1987), Valentino *et al.* (1987), Lewis *et al.* (1988, 1989), Baldino *et al.* (1989), Eakin *et al.* (1994), Brimijoin *et al.* (1996), Chabot *et al.* (1996), and Jonker *et al.* (1997).

Tissue preparation and fixation

Tissue should be snap frozen as rapidly as possible (for example, by using isopentane cooled to the temperature of liquid nitrogen) before mounting on cryostat chucks and cutting of sections using a cryostat microtome. Sections are thaw mounted on to microscope slides that have been heated to 180 °C overnight to destroy RNase and coated with APES (3-aminopropyltriethoxy-silane); gelatin, albumen, and poly-L-lysine have also been used instead of APES. For quantitative assays, it is essential to ensure that tissue sections are cut to reproducible and uniform thickness. Section thickness can vary with the speed of cutting which can be reduced by using a motor-driven microtome. For ^{35}S-labelled oligonucleotide probes, a linear relationship has been demonstrated between section thickness (range 5–25 μm) and the amount of specific probe hybridization. This would be expected since increasing the section thickness increases the total RNA per unit area and suggests that there are no barriers to the penetration of the probe (Nunez *et al.* 1989). Typically, 10 μm thick sections are used, although Singer *et al.* (1987) recommend 5 μm to improve resolution, but these can be more difficult to cut routinely using a cryostat microtome.

Fixation is a critical step in performing quantitative assays in order to prevent the loss of mRNA from tissue sections and preserve tissue morphology. Messenger RNA must be immobilized without introducing barriers to the penetration of the probe. The aim is to fix tissue (for example, from control and experimental animals) under the same conditions. This can be difficult if tissue is fixed prior to cutting. Fixation after cutting sections is recommended as this can be more carefully controlled: as a guide, for 5–30 min in a freshly prepared solution of 4% formaldehyde in phosphate-buffered saline (0.05 M, pH 7.4). This is based on detailed comparisons of fixatives for *in situ* hybridization made by Lawrence and Singer (1985) and Singer *et al.* (1987). Formaldehyde is the optimal fixative, as the cytosol is cross-linked to give good tissue preservation but the mRNA is still accessible for hybridization. Glutaraldehyde tends to cause more extensive cross-linking of proteins. A permeabilization step using acids, proteases, or detergents may be required (Singer *et al.* 1987), but this can cause variable loss of mRNA from the tissue and this step should be avoided for quantitative assays. Loss of tissue mRNA by RNases should be minimized by wearing gloves at all times.

Choice of probes

Three types of probe are commonly used. For quantitative *in situ* hybridization, single-stranded oligonucleotide probes (usually 15–50 bases) can be easily prepared using a DNA synthesizer. An advantage is that there are no barriers to penetration of the probe into tissue sections up to 25 μm thick (Nunez *et al.* 1989). However, these probes may form less stable hybrids. More complex cloning methods or the polymerase chain reaction are used to produce complementary DNA (cDNA) probes. Large cRNAs may be derived from cDNAs that have been cloned into appropriate plasmids, but small cRNA molecules can be made on synthetic DNA templates (see Chapters 3 and 4).

Choice of isotope

A number of isotopes have been used to label probes for *in situ* hybridization. These isotopes are ranked in Table 5.1 according to the energy of their emitted particles, starting with the highest, ^{32}P. Probes can be labelled to high specific activity with this isotope, Allowing autoradiograms to be produced

Table 5.1 Characterisitics of isotopes used to label probes

	^{32}P	^{33}P	^{35}S	^{125}I	^{3}H
Half-life	14 days β-	25 days β-	87 days β-	60 days Electron capture	12.3 years β-
Maximum specific activity (Ci/mg)	285.5	156.2	42.7	17.5	9.6
Maximum particle energy (keV)	1710	249	167		19
Mean particle energy (keV)	690 690		49	3 (28%)* 4 (49%) 23 (14%) 31 (7%) 34 (1%)	5.7
Detection					
Film type	β-Max	β-Max	β-Max	β-Max	^{3}H
Film resolution	Low	Medium	Medium	High	High
Exposure time	Rapid	Rapid	Medium	Medium	Long
Polymer standards		^{14}C	^{14}C	^{125}I	^{3}H

* ^{125}I emits extranuclear electrons with the indicated discrete energies. The proportion is given in parentheses (Rogers 1979). Autoradiography films (Hyperfilm β-Max and Hyperfilm ^{3}H), and ^{14}C, ^{3}H, and ^{125}I polymer standards are supplied by Amersham International plc, Amersham, Bucks, UK.

within hours or a few days. For quantitative assays, a disadvantage is that owing to the short half-life of this isotope, standards (which are not commercially available) must be prepared frequently. The maximum emission energy of 33^P is lower than ^{32}P, producing better autoradiographical resolution although the half-life is still comparatively short. Sulfur-35 is the most widely used of these three isotopes for quantitative assays and is the label of choice, producing clear macro-autoradiograms with good resolution and it has the longest half-life. Tritium-labelled probes give the highest resolution. However, owing to the lower specific activities of the probes, exposure times of several months may be required. Higher specific activities are possible using ^{125}I and this isotope is extensively used to label ligands for receptor autoradiography (Davenport *et al.* 1988). Resolution can be as good as tritium, since extranuclear electrons and not the γ-rays contribute to the formation of the autoradiographical image. This isotope has not been widely used to label probes and its use in quantitative assays has not been evaluated.

In situ hybridization assays: determining optimum probe concentrations

The hybridization step is to provide optimal conditions for the formation of hybrids between the labelled oligonucleotide and the target nucleic acid. The conditions of hybridization are varied to give the appropriate stringency. For quantitative assays it is important to ensure that the labelled probe is present in excess of the target nucleotide sequence. This can be determined by adding increasing amounts of the labelled probe in a fixed volume of buffer to adjacent, consecutive sections of tissue. There should be a linear relationship between probe concentration and the amount of probe hybridized until a plateau is observed. At this point, the probe is saturating all available hybridization sites in the tissue. Subsequent quantitative assays should use concentrations well above this value, so that experiments performed at different times can be compared (Nunez *et al.* 1989). When the probe is present in excess over the tissue mRNA concentration, the reaction is thought to follow pseudo-first-order kinetics (Tecott *et al.* 1987). Some indication of the optimal time for incubation can be calculated based on the length, concentration and probe complexity (see Tecott, *et al.* 1987) but, in practice, most assays are left overnight with high probe concentration and there is little advantage in extending the time beyond 16 h (Angerer *et al.* 1981).

Measurement of non-specific hybridization

Radiolabelled probes may bind non-specifically to proteins, polysaccharides, and nucleic acids in the tissue sections. This can be reduced, but rarely eliminated, by adding a range of blocking compounds to the pre-hybridization buffer. For oligonucleotide probes, a convenient method of estimating non-specific hybridization is to treat adjacent sections of tissue for 30 min at 37°C with a solution (100 μg/ml) of RNase in 0.5 NTE enzyme buffer (10 mM Tris, 0.5 M NaCl, 1 mM EDTA, pH 8) previously boiled to destroy DNase activity. The sections are then incubated for a further 30 min in the buffer alone. At the concentration of RNase employed, it is expected that all single-stranded RNA species are cleaved and are, therefore, unavailable for hybridization.

For RNA probes, the corresponding sense probe can be synthesized and labelled to the same specific activity as the antisense probe. Theoretically, none of these probes, when labelled, should hybridize to the tissue; any binding to the sections is non-specific and gives a measure of the general 'stickiness' of the probe. This may reveal any usual probe-binding properties of a particular tissue (see, for example, Nunez *et al.* 1990).

Autoradiography

Following *in situ* hybridization, the dry slides are securely mounted to rigid board using adhesive tape to prevent movement, and are placed in a light-tight X-ray cassette. For quantitative autoradiography, high resolution films that have a single layer of emulsion coated on to a transparent polyester base, such as Hyperfilm β Max (Amersham International plc) are recommended for ^{35}S, ^{33}P, ^{32}P, and ^{125}I. Hyperfilm ^{3}H, which lacks the anti-abrasive layer, is used to detect ^{3}H and can be used for ^{125}I isotopes. Up to 64 slides including standards can be apposed at the same time using the largest size of Hyperfilm β Max (35 cm × 43 cm). Potential errors that can arise in detecting radio-activity with the film are discussed by Davenport *et al.* (1988, 1989). These can be reduced by ensuring slides bearing replicate sections are positioned throughout the area occupied by the film.

At the end of the exposure, films are manually developed using a con-ventional developer such as Kodak D-19 for 3 min at 17°C with intermittent agitation, rinsed for 30 sec in deionized water, and fixed for 5 min at 20°C. Films are washed (for at least 15 min) and dried. All procedures should be carried out in total darkness or with minimal exposure to red safelight (Kodak Wratten 6B or equivalent) to monitor the progress of development.

Preparation of standards

Calibrated radioactive standards are conveniently prepared by mixing increasing quantities of the radionuclide to be quantified with tissue paste (usually from rat brain) in microcentrifuge tubes (Davenport and Hall, 1988). In order to obtain a suitable range of optical density values in the resulting autoradiographical image when apposed to radiation-sensitive film, a mini-mum of about eight standards with different activity levels should be prepared by constructing a dilution curve as follows: 1, 0.66, 0.50, 0.33, 0.25, 0.17, 0.12,

0.06. The concentration of radioactivity selected for the initial solution will depend on the anticipated length of exposure. This will be influenced mainly by the energy of the radionuclide and the specific activity of the probe (Table 5.1). For example, in order to produce standards 10 μm thick for the quantification of ^{35}S oligonucleotides within autoradiographical images produced by exposing cardiovascular or neuronal tissue to Hyperfilm β-max for 1–14 days, the initial solution in the dilution series contains about 10 μCi of radioactivity, which is added to 650 mg of tissue. Cryostat sections are cut from the frozen cylinders to the same thickness as the experimental sections and the amount of radioactivity in each section is measured by scintillation counting in dpm, having made appropriate corrections for background and the efficiency of counting.

Polymer standards

Commercial standards are available (Amersham International plc) for ^{3}H (high activity range 3–110 nCi/mg) and ^{125}I (activity range 2–640 nCi/mg). They consist of layers containing radioactivity incorporated at the molecular level in a methacrylate copolymer, separated by inert coloured layers. Standards are available in pre-cut strips, or as a multilayer block from which sections can be cut on a rotary microtome. Cut strips are expanded on water at 60°C and brushed flat on to gelatin-subbed slides to remove creases. Representative sections are subdivided into the individual activity levels and counted as described above.

Ideally, standards should be prepared from the same isotope as that used to label the probe. However, polymer standards are not available for ^{35}S (Table 5.1). The average energy of the β-particles emitted by ^{14}C is the same as ^{35}S (49 keV) although the maximum energy (156 keV) is slightly lower. The slopes of calibration curves produced by ^{14}C polymer and ^{35}35 tissue paste standards are not significantly different. Therefore, ^{14}C polymer standards can be used to quantify ^{35}S-labelled probes in tissue sections, although a correction factor should be determined if absolute amounts of radioactivity are required. Carbon-14 standards with two ranges of specific activity are available. The highest specific activity (30–880 nCi/mg) is recommended, giving a set of standards ranging from 120 to 1300 dpm. With a high-life of 5730 years, decay of the standards will not be significant. These standards have also been used to calibrate ^{33}P tissue paste standards using Hyperfilm β-Max film from 1–14 days exposure (Eakin *et al.* 1994).

Computer-assisted image analysis

The resulting autoradiograms are analysed by measuring diffuse integrated optical density using a computer-assisted image analysis system. A range of image analysers are available, but in order to carry out accurate densitometry the machine should be equipped with a shading corrector (ideally with the correction performed in real-time before each scan) and should be able to digitize images into an array of at least 500 × 500 picture points, with a minimum of 256 grey levels. The image analyser should also be able to subtract stored images. The details of operation of different commercial systems vary considerably, but the major procedures are similar, and can be illustrated using the Quantimet 970 (Leica UK Ltd, Milton Keynes, UK), which uses a computer program developed for quantitative autoradiography (Davenport *et al.* 1988, 1989).

Autoradiograms are illuminated by reflected white light and the image is captured by the video scanner equipped with a zoom lens. Each image is digitized into an array of 630 000 image points each with a grey value in the range 0–255. Once captured, the operator can manipulate the images presented on a high-resolution monitor using a digitablet with a hand-operated cursor and an alphanumeric keyboard.

The image analyser is first calibrated for densitometry. This should be repeated each time the conditions are changed, such as altering the magnification or using a different film. The zoom lens mounted on the video scanner is altered to produce a measuring field appropriate to the size of the autoradiographical image. The shading corrector is set to give an image that appears uniformly white and compensates for any variation in illumination so that optical densities can be measured accurately throughout the autoradiogram. The white level (100% transmission) is set and the scanner dark current (the current flowing in the scanner in the absence of a signal), which would otherwise contribute to the grey image, is eliminated. Finally, the system is calibrated against neutral density filters to convert grey levels into optical densities and the number of pixels per unit area is calculated by means of a measuring box.

Constructing a standard curve from calibrated standards

A standard curve is constructed for each film to relate optical densities to known amounts of radioactivity. The autoradiographical image of each standard is detected and the cursor used to draw around and isolate the image. The integrated optical density for each standard, together with the area, is determined. The radioactivity of each standard, measured by liquid scintillation counting, is then divided by the area to calculate radioactivity in dpm/mm^2. The image analyser generates a natural log plot of optical density versus radioactivity which gives a linear relationship (Fig. 5.1).

The concentration of probe hybridizing to tissue sections is measured by digitizing each autoradiographical image of tissue sections. The operator can select regions of interest from the resulting grey image displayed on a high resolution monitor by using a cursor to draw around a defined anatomical region. Other binary masks in the form of circles or boxes can be used to

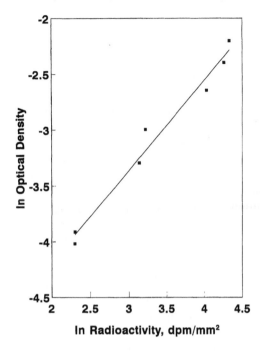

Fig. 5.1. An example of a natural log plot of optical density versus radioactivity for ^{35}S tissue paste standards exposed directly to Hyperfilm β-Max film. (Each value represents the mean of three determinations. Standard errors were less than 3% of the mean.)

sample from within a structure. The computer isolates the areas defined by these masks and measures the integrated optical density. When all measurements have been made the threshold for detecting the autoradiogram is increased to produce a template, which is used to align the autoradiographical image of an adjacent section treated either with RNase or control sense probe. The second image is digitally subtracted from the first to obtain a new image of the specific hybridization of the probe. Optical densities are converted to radioactivity values by interpolation from the standards curve and these values are then divided by the specific activity of the probe to calculate the amount of probe specifically hybridized to each structure, in moles per unit area.

Corrections are made for any decay of the labelled probe (particularly important for ^{32}P and ^{33}P) from the time at which these measurements were made to the midpoint between apposing and developing the film. Since standards are used repeatedly (with the exception of ^{14}C), the radioactive content should be corrected for decay from the date when they were counted and the midpoint between apposing and developing the film.

The relationship between film optical density and tissue radioactivity may vary as a result of various factors, including the characteristics of the radiation source, the type of emulsion, the conditions of exposure, and the method of development. A number of mathematical transformations have been used to describe this relationship. One approach is to use a natural log plot of optical density versus radioactivity to give a linear relationship, as shown in Fig. 5.1 for a series of ^{35}S tissue paste standards apposed to Hyperfilm β-Max. However, both Hyperfilm ^{3}H and β-Max rapidly approach saturation at an optical density of one (Davenport and Hall, 1988). At this point increases in radioactivity result in little or no increase in optical density and the linear relationship will be lost. The upper and lower limits for making accurate measurements for each type of film and image analyser should be determined. Using the Quantimet to analyse Hyperfilm β-Max, variation in optical densities of less than 5% are obtained within the linear range 0.1–0.8. Ideally, tissue sections should be exposed to produce optical density values falling within this range and can be reapposed where necessary. The majority of factors that affect the response of emulsions to radioactivity are therefore controlled for by co-exposing calibrated standards with each film and generating an appropriate curve. The inter- and intra-assay coefficients of variation using *in situ* hybridization and quantitative autoradiography to measure tissue RNA have been estimated to be less than 10 and 7%, respectively (Nunez *et al.* 1989). This compares with an inter-assay variation using micro-autoradiography as the detection system of 25–30% (McCabe *et al.* 1986).

Application of quantitative *in situ* hybridization

Measurement of peptide mRNA by ^{35}S-labelled oligonucleotide probes

An example of quantifying mRNA in tissue sections using a ^{35}S-labelled oligonucleotide probe to investigate alterations in gene expression of a peptide is shown in Fig. 5.2. A 42-mer probe [complementary to atrial natriuretic factor (ANF) mRNA sequence coding for pro-ANF 103–116] was used to localize and measure changes in mRNA produced by mineralo-corticoid/saline treatment in sections of rat heart (Nunez *et al.* 1989). Measurements were made on autoradiographical images showing the total amount of probe hybridized. The image of an adjacent section treated with RNase was digitally subtracted from the first and the amount of probe specifically hybridized to the heart was calculated in amol/mm^2 by interpolation from the previously generated standards curve. Figure 5.2 shows that the amount of probe hybridized to adult hearts from the control was significantly lower in the left or right atria, as well as in the ventricle, compared with the saline/deoxycortisone-treated rats.

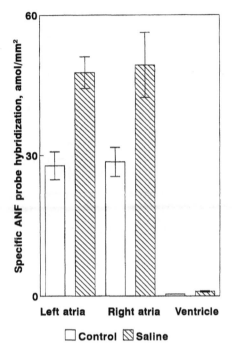

Fig. 5.2. Quantification of tissue mRNA using a ^{35}S-labelled oligonucleotide probe. The results show the amount of specific hybridization of a 3′-end-labelled ANF mRNA probe to adult heart removed from control or saline/deoxycortisone-treated rats. The levels of ANF mRNA probe binding in atria and ventricles were significantly elevated in the saline/mineralocorticoid-treated rats compared with the control. Each value represents the mean of 12 determinations ± sem. (From Nunez *et al.* 1989.)

Measurement of receptor mRNA by ^{35}S-labelled RNA probes

Examples of the use of ^{35}S-labelled RNA probes to compare the distribution of mRNA encoding the two endothelin receptor subtypes, ET_A and ET_B, in sections of human cardiac tissue are shown in Figs 5.3–5.5. It was previously thought that smooth muscle cells of blood vessels only express ET_A receptors, whereas the ET_B subtype was localized to the vascular endothelium. Quantitative autoradiography was used to measure levels of mRNA encoding both receptors in the media (smooth muscle layer) of epicardial coronary arteries as well as the smaller intramyocardial vessels within heart muscle.

ET_A (bases 439–737) and ET_B (bases 497–924) polymerase chain reaction-amplified DNA bands were cloned into pBluescript II KS and the linearized inserts used as templates to generate ^{35}S-labelled antisense and sense (control) RNA probes. The resulting autoradiographical images showing the distribution and density of hybridization of the two probes and their corresponding controls in adjacent sections is shown in Fig. 5.3 for cross-

In situ *Hybridization*

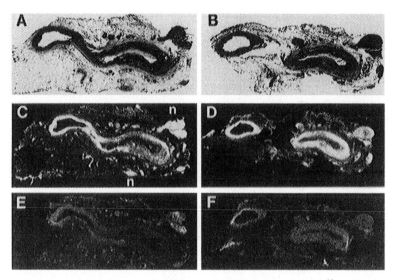

Fig. 5.3. Autoradiographical images showing the distribution of antisense ^{35}S-labelled probes for endothelin ET_A (C) and ET_B (D) mRNA in coronal sections of human epicardial coronary artery. Adjacent sections were incubated with the corresponding sense control probes labelled to the same specific activity and are shown in (E) and (F), respectively. This gives a measure of the non-specific binding of the probes. (A) and (B) are bright-field micrographs of haematoxylin and eosin sections (n = nerves). (Modified from Davenport *et al.* 1993.)

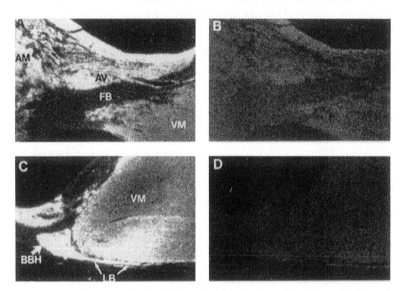

Fig. 5.4. Autoradiograhical images showing the distribution of antisense (A, C) and sense control probe in adjacent sections (B,D) for endothelin ET_A receptor mRNA in human heart. (A) Atrioventricular node (AV) and (C) branching bundle of His (BBH), left bundle branch (LB), ventricular (VM), and atrial myocardium (AM). Messenger RNA was localized to all areas of the heart excluding the central fibrous body (FB). (Modified from Molenaar *et al.* 1993.)

82

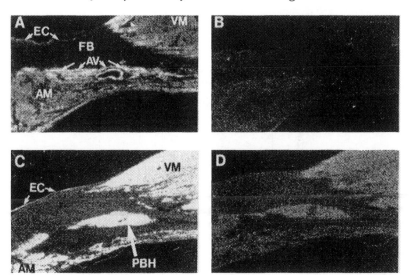

Fig. 5.5. Autoradiographical images showing the distribution of antisense (A,C) and sense control probe for ET$_B$ receptor mRNA (B,D) in human heart. (A) Atrioventricular node and (B) penetrating bundle of His. Abbreviations are the same as in Fig. 5.4. Messenger RNA was also localized to all areas of the heart excluding the central fibrous body (FB). (Modified from Molenaar *et al.* 1993.)

sections of epicardial coronary arteries and in the conducting system of the heart (Figs 5.4 and 5.5). Quantitative autoradiography was used to compare the amount of probe specifically hybridizing to epicardial arteries compared with the intramyocardial resistance vessels (Fig. 5.6) by digitally subtracting the autoradiographical image of the sense control probe from that of the antisense probe (Davenport *et al.* 1993, 1995; Molenaar *et al.* 1993). The results show similar amounts of probe for both receptors hybridized to the intramyocardial vessels, whereas mRNA encoding the ET$_A$ subtype predominated in the epicardial arteries. Since ET$_B$ mRNA was also widely distributed in cardiac muscle, *in situ* hybridization was required to isolate and measure the amounts of ET$_B$ message present in blood vessels within this tissue.

Conclusions

With careful selection of the isotope and design of the assay conditions, *in situ* hybridization and macro-autoradiography can be used to measure changes in gene expression in tissue sections. Detection of radiolabelled probes by autoradiography continues to be one of the most sensitive methods for visualizing mRNA and is most reproducible when inter-assay variability is controlled by the use of radioactive reference standards. The technique is particularly powerful where the anatomical structure of tissue must be preserved in order to quantify mRNA in discrete regions.

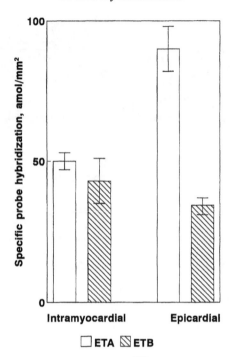

Fig. 5.6. Quantification of tissue mRNA using a ^{35}S-labelled RNA probe. The results show the amount of specific hybridization of ET_A and ET_B probes measured in the media (smooth muscle layer) of epicardial coronary arteries shown in Fig. 5.3 and intramyocardial vessels (Figs 5.4 and 5.5). Each value is the mean ± sem of three individuals. In each case, the amount of probe specifically hybridized was determined by digitally subtracting the autoradiographical images (shown in Figs 5.3–5.5) of the sense control probe from that of the antisense probe using computer-assisted densitometry. (Davenport *et al.* 1995.)

Acknowledgements

This work was supported by grants from the British Heart Foundation, the Royal Society, and the Isaac Newton Trust.

References

Angerer, L.M. and Angerer, R.C. (1981). Detection of poly A [+]RNA in sea urchin eggs and embryos by quantitative *in situ* hybridization. *Nucl. Acids Res.*, **9**, 2819–40.

Baubet, V., Fevre Montange, M., Gay, N., Debilly, G., Bobillier, P., and Cespuglio, R. (1994). Effects of an acute immobilization stress upon proopiomelanocortin (POMC) mRNA levels in the mediobasal hypoethalamus: a quantitative *in situ* hybridization study. *Mol. Brain Res.*, **26**, 163–8.

Baldino, F., Chesselet, M-F., and Lewis, M.E. (1989). High resolution *in situ* hybridization histochemistry. *Meth. Enzymol.*, **168**, 761–77.

Brimijoin, S. and Hammond, P. (1996). Transient expression of acetylcholinesterase messenger RNA and enzyme activity in developing rat thalamus studied by quantitative histochemistry and *in situ* hybridization. *Neuroscience*, **71**, 555–65.

Chabot, J.G., Kar, S., and Quirion, R.T.I. (1996). Autoradiographical and immunohistochemical analysis of receptor localization in the central nervous system. *Histochem. J.*, **28**, 729–45.

Davneport, A.P. and Hall, M.D. (1988). Comparison between brain paste and polymer [^{125}I] standards for quantitative receptor autoradiography. *J. Neurosci. Meth.*, **25**, 75–82.

Davenport, A.P., Beresford, I.J.M., Hall, M.D., Hill, R.G., and Hughes, J. (1988). Quantitative autoradiography in neuroscience. In: *Molecular neuroanatomy*, (ed. F.W. Van Leeuwen, R.M. Buijs, C.W. Pool and O. Pach), pp. 121–45. Elsevier, Amsterdam.

Davenport, A.P., Hill, R.G., and Hughes, J. (1989). Quantitative analysis of autoradiograms. In: *Regulatory peptides*, (ed. J. Polak, pp. 137–53. Birkhauser, Basel.

Davenport, A.P., O'Reilly, G., Molenaar, P., Maguire, J.J., Kuc, R.E., Sharkey, A., Bacon, C.R., and Ferro, A. (1993). Human endothelin receptors characterised using reverse transcriptase-polymerase chain reaction, *in situ* hybridization and sub-type selective ligands BQ123 and BQ3020: evidence for expression of ET$_B$ receptors in human vascular smooth muscle. *J. Cardiovasc. Pharmacol.*, **22**(S8), 22–5.

Davenport, A.P., O'Reilly, G., and Kuc, R.E. (1995). Endothelin ET$_A$ and ET$_B$ mRNA and receptors are expressed by smooth muscle in the human vasculature, but the ET$_A$ sub-type predominates. *Br. J. Pharmacol.*, **114**, 1110–16.

Eakin, T.J., Baskin, D.G., Breininger, J.F., and Stahl, W.L. (1994). Calibration of ^{14}C standards for quantitative autoradiography with ^{33}P. *J. Histochem. Cytochem.*, **42**, 1295–8.

Eastwood, S.L., Burnet, P.W.J., McDonald, B., Clinton, J., and Harrison, P.J. (1994). Synaptophysin gene expression in human brain: a quantitative *in situ* hybridization and immunocytochemical study. *Neuroscience*, **59**, 881–92.

Jonker, A., de Boer, P.A., van den Hoff, M.J., Lamers, W.H., and Moorman, A.F. (1997). Towards quantitative *in situ* hybridization. *J. Histochem.* Cytochem., **45**, 413–23.

Lawrence, J.B. and Singer, R.H. (1985). Quantitative analysis of *in situ* hybridization methods for the detection of actin gene expression. *Nucl. Acids Res.*, **13**, 1777–99.

Lewis, M.E., Krause, R.G., and Robert-Lewis, J.M. (1988). Recent developments in the use of synthetic oligonucleotides for *in situ* hybridization histochemistry. *Synapse*, **2**, 308–16.

Lewis, M.E., Rogers, W.T., Krause, R.G., and Schwaber, J.S. (1989). Quantitation and digital representation of *in situ* hybridization histochemistry. *Meth. Enzymol.*, **168**, 808–21.

McCabe, J.T., Morrell, J.I., Richter, D., and Pfaff, D.W. (1986). Localization of neuroendocrinologically relevant RNA in brain by *in situ* hybridization. *Front. Neuroendocrinol.*, **9**, 149–67.

Molenaar, P., P.Reilly, G., Sharkey, A., Kuc, R.E., Harding, D.P., Plumpton, P., Gresham, G.A., and Davenport, A.P. (1993). Characterization and localization of endothelin receptor sub-types in the human atioventricular conducting system and myocardium. *Circul. Res.*, **72**, 526–38.

Nunez, D.J., Davenport, A.P., Emson, P.C., and Brown, M.J. (1989). A quntitative 'in-situ' hybridization method using computer-assisted image analysis. Validation and measurement of Atrial Natriuretic Factor (ANF) messenger RNA in the rat heart. *Biochem. J.*, **263**, 121–7.

Nunez, D.J., Davenport, A.P., and Brown, M.J. (1990). Atrial natriuretic factor messenger RNA and binding sites in the adrenal gland. *Biochem. J.*, **271**, 555–8.

Penschow, J.D., Haralambidis, P.E., Darling, P.E., Darby, I.A., Wintour, E.M., Tregear, G.W., and Coghlan, J.P. (1987). Hybridization histochemistry. *Experientia*, **43**, 741–9.

Radja, F., El Mansari, M., Soghomonian, J.J., Dewar, K.M., Ferron, A., Reader, T.A., and Descarries, L. (1993). Changes of D1 and D2 receptors in adult rat neostriatum after neonatal dopamine denervation: quantitative data from ligand binding, *in situ* hybridization and iontophoresis. *Neuroscience*, **57**, 635–48.

Rogers, A.W. (1979). *Techniques of autoradiography*, 3rd edn. Elsevier, Amsterdam.

Singer, R.H., Lawrence, J.B., and Rashtchian, R.N. (1987). Towards a rapid and sensitive *in situ* hybridization methodology using isotopic and nonisotopic probes. In: *In situ* hybridization: applications to neurobiology, (eds. K.L. Valentino, J.H. Erberwine, and J.D. Barchus), pp. 71–96. Oxford University Press, New York.

Tecott, L.H., Eberwine, J.H., Barchas, J.D., and Valentino, K.L. (1987). Methodological considerations in the utilization of *in situ* hybridization. In: *In situ hybridization: applications to neurobiology*, (ed. K.L. Valentino, J.H. Erberwine, and J.D. Barchus), pp. 1–23. Oxford University Press, New York.

Tracer, H.L. and Loh, Y.P. (1993). The effect of salt-loading on corticotropin releasing hormone and arginine vasopressin mRNA levels in the mouse hypothalamus: a quantitative *in situ* hybridization analysis. *Neuropeptides*, **25**, 161–7.

Valentino, K.L., Erberwine, J.H., and Barchus, J.D. (ed.) (1987). In: *In situ hybridization: applications to neurobiology*. Oxford University Press, New York.

Young, W.S. and Kuhar, M.J. (1986). Quantitative *in situ* hybridization and determination of mRNA content. In: *In situ hybridization in Brain*, (ed. G.R. Uhl, pp. 245–8. Plenum Press, New York.

6

Quantification of grains in *in situ* hybridization

JANE ALDRIDGE

Image analysis provides a wide range of sophisticated measurement techniques. Even so, it is often difficult to analyse histological and cytological preparations automatically since, in many cases, standard detection methods simply do not interpret the image well enough on their own to find the regions to be measured. This is particularly true for radiolabelled *in situ* hybridization. The issue of recognition is complex, since the best approach to interpreting an image automatically often depends on background information about the sample and about the aims of the experiment. Important changes in the approach adopted by manufacturers of image analysis equipment are promising advances. The first is a shift away from developing general analysis software and towards developing analysis software that will solve particular problems in interpreting types of images. The second is a realization that image analysis is only the end-point of a wider experiment, and that contextual information should be taken into account when designing the image analysis experiment.

In this chapter, a new software package for cellular level quantification of grains in *in situ* hybridization is described which was developed by Seescan plc (Cambridge) and is now commercially available. This package is novel in that it is not simply an adaptation of general purpose image analysis tools, but instead employs pattern recognition algorithms that were developed especially for this application and extensively validated to form the basis of the interpretation process.

The binding sites of radiolabelled mRNA transcripts in *in situ* hybridization and ligands in receptor autoradiography studies can be localized to the cellular level if the appropriate radioactive isotope is used. The results of binding are normally visualized by apposing a coverslip coated with a photographic emulsion to the section, because it is easier to achieve an even coating of emulsion on a coverslip than by the alternative technique of dipping the section into photographic emulsion. After a period of exposure, the emulsion is developed. Where levels of radioactivity in the section are higher than a minimum, grains of silver halide form in the emulsion layer. Sections have usually first been counterstained to reveal the histological structure of the sample so the silver halide grains are seen superimposed on the counterstained cells using bright-field microscopy at an appropriate magnification.

Low levels of labelling can be easily assessed by eye, simply by counting the numbers of silver halide grains superimposed on a single cell or on groups of cells. When grains become more dense, clumping occurs, and clumps are hard to assess visually. However, even at low levels, the sheer volume of grain counting needed in many experiments to generate statistically valid data is daunting if the work has to be done by eye.

The minimum specification of image analysis hardware required for quantifying grains is a high resolution monochrome camera normally mounted using a 'C' mount on to the microscope, a monitor on which to see the image it produces, and a framestore to capture digitally the image sensed by the camera. The framestore must be accessible by an appropriate processor capable of running the quantification software.

Attempts to use automatic image analysis to quantify the extent of radio-labelling on counterstained sections have, in the past, been confounded by the difficulty of thresholding the grains. Thresholding is a common method used in image analysis to detect the features of interest in the image. In an ideal world, the user would be able to select a particular grey shade that was darker than all of the counterstained cells, and lighter than all of the grains. Although the grains are easy to see visually, a threshold level that detects grains on lightly counterstained regions of the image will usually overdetect grains on heavily counterstained cells, and will often even detect the cells themselves. This phenomenon is thought to be caused by optical diffraction effects resulting from the small (submicrometre) size of individual grains, and by video bandwidth limitations arising from basic camera design and from filtering the video at the input to the image analysis system to meet Nyquist's theorem. A further problem arises from the relative thickness of the sample. At the highest magnifications, it is not normally possible to select a single focal plane in which both the counterstained cells and the grains are adequately focused. In fact, the thickness of the emulsion layer in which grains can form is often greater than the depth of focus at high magnifications.

Two analysis methods had previously been developed to overcome some of the problems and to enable automatic image analysis to be used to quantify grain density. The first method uses dark field microscopy. The counterstain information disappears from the image, while the grains appear as bright dots on a black background. This technique is commonly used in receptor autoradiography and *in situ* hybridization. Its main disadvantage is that grain density can no longer be related to histological structure unless the bright-field image is also referred to, involving swapping regularly between dark-field and bright-field images of the same field of view.

In the second method, the section is counterstained so lightly that a single threshold can be chosen which properly detects all grains and does not pick up the counterstain. This technique is commonly used in the unscheduled DNA synthesis assay for assessing chemical compounds for genetic toxicity. The disadvantage is that, in practice, the counterstain often proves so light that it can be difficult to make out the histological structure of the sample. Moreover, to avoid problems of video bandwidth limitations hindering thresholding, analyses are normally performed using a $\times 100$ oil immersion objective, which results in the need to change the plane of focus regularly and analyse multiple fields of view. In many autoradiographic applications, this would slow down analysis considerably. Moreover, this method is particularly unsuitable for tissues that counterstain non-homogeneously.

It is desirable to quantify radiolabelling on bright-field images of samples that have been counterstained to make their morphology easy to recognize and at magnifications that give the maximum depth of focus while allowing grains to be well resolved. For this reason, Seescan made the following assumptions and used these to form the basis of the rule set from which it started to develop its quantification package.

First, the silver halide grains would be as well focused as possible and the magnification would be set so that single grains were as small as possible on the screen, commensurate with their being well resolved. Secondly, the counterstained cells would tend to be less well focused than the grains. Thirdly, there would be a contrast difference between grains and their local background. Fourthly, unless there were large clumps of grains, the size of counterstained objects would be significantly larger than the size of grains. Finally, grains would either be single or clumped.

Software was developed that detected single grains, and small and large clumps of grains using pattern recognition techniques and relative density information and which would work on images captured using either a $\times 20$ or $\times 40$ objective, the choice depending on the grain size. The software was optimized by checking its results using a routine which, on a key press, switched on or off a yellow or green overlay superimposed on the image to show the results of the detection over the original image.

An early observation was that it is necessary for the user to be able to vary the severity with which algorithms are applied to adapt for different grain sizes. The problem of assessing clumps was addressed by measuring the total area covered by grains within a region of interest, and then expressing the grain cover either per unit area or per cell. A count estimate was derived for comparison with visual counts by dividing the area of grain cover by the average area of a single grain.

Initial studies showed that these algorithms gave better than 99% repeatability on the same image, and also showed that the data were significantly more immune to variations in lighting than data produced by the standard method involving quantifying the dark field image. Dr Jonathan Seckl's team at the University of Edinburgh performed validation studies comparing the data acquired automatically with counts made by eye. At low densities, a correlation of 98% was reported. At higher densities the correlation was not so good; 87% was reported. This was thought to be because the difficulty of assessing grain density visually increases as the labelling becomes heavier. Tests were performed using commercially available ^{32}P and ^{35}S standards (Amersham, Hemel Hempstead) apposed to emulsion-coated coverslips. A 97% correlation was shown between the nominal radioactivity values of the standards and the grain densities measured using the new techniques. It was felt that this indication the validity of the measurement technique and that it supported the hypothesis that at higher densities visual assessment is less accurate than automatic assessment. The graph of nominal versus measured values also shows the start of the typical non-linearity at higher radioactivity levels experienced in autoradiography owing to saturation of the emulsion. These methods were shown to give a time improvement of about 10 times over visual analysis.

A user friendly software program was written using these algorithms specifically for *in situ* hybridization and receptor autoradiography. It allows the operator to set up and execute an experiment by defining and then implementing a protocol. In the protocol definition, the user describes the experiment, including identifying the sections to be analysed and the regions to be analysed for each section. During the protocol set-up the grain detection algorithms are optimized on experimental and control samples, and will then be applied identically to all samples throughout the experiment. The user can specify whether grain density should be assessed per cell or per unit area, and how data are to be corrected, if at all, for variations in background labelling. A range of calibration algorithms can be used to convert image analysis data to the units used in calibration standards if this is required.

During the analysis, the operator presents new fields of view to the image analyser, having first identified the section and the anatomical region to be analysed. The image analyser finds the grains automatically using the special image-processing algorithms at the severity set up in the protocol. The user can then outline cells or anatomical structures using circular and rectangular frames of variable size and shape, or by drawing around them freehand. The area defined by the user is measured automatically and reported in calibrated units along with grain cover, i.e. the area covered by grains within the region defined by the user and which has been shown to be equivalent to the grain count. At this stage, the user can define the number of cells that have just been analysed, so that data may be presented on a per area or per cell basis. Although data are normally reported as average results for anatomical regions on a per section basis, it is possible to access each raw data point, and, if images are being stored of each field of view that is analysed, for each data point, the image with the area from which the measurement was taken can be reviewed, thus providing a full audit trail through the experiment.

This software has now been used successfully for a number of studies

(Mohammed *et al.* 1993; Farman *et al.* 1994; Olsson *et al.* 1994; Yau *et al.* 1994) and is gaining wide acceptance. Although originally written for Seescan's own image analysers, the software has been recoded to operate within the PC Windows environment and can be used with images captured using non-Seescan hardware. As the algorithms are relatively tolerant of variation in absolute grey level representation, data are unlikely to be significantly worsened by using less accurate image capture systems than those supplied by Seescan. OLE programming structures have been used so that data generated can be transferred to and manipulated within Excel, and then copied to word-processing packages.

It is important that consistency is observed in sample preparation and analysis, particularly regarding factors such as section thickness and the methods adopted for defining the regions of analysis. This program allows sensitive comparisons to be made between experimental samples and controls, but because of artefacts largely resulting from sectioning, in which a cell may be bisected, thus losing some of its mRNA, it cannot, other than through the use of properly prepared calibration standards, be used to generate truly accurate data about the number of grains formed per complete cell within a structure. Methods have been published (McCabe and Bolender 1993) based on stereological techniques that claim to provide these data. However, they are significantly more cumbersome at providing the type of comparative data that this package can generate.

In developing this package it was noted that for quantitation, significantly better results will be obtained by using emulsion-coated coverslips rather than by dipping the sections in emulsion. This is because a fundamental and necessary assumption in quantitiation is that the thickness of the emulsion layer will not vary significantly within a relatively large area of the section to ensure that the number of grains that will form within a region, owing to a fixed amount of radioactivity, is constant. As tissue processing often results in sections having uneven surfaces, with hollows, it is difficult to guarantee even coating with dipped sections. A further disadvantage of working with dipped sections is that the grains are likely to go in and out of focus as the topology of the surface changes, and this can be exasperating as it may be necessary to work at several different focal levels to analyse fully all of the cells within a single field of view.

References

Farman, N., Bonvalet, J.-P., and Seckl, J.R. (1994). Aldosterone selectively increases Na$^+$, K$^+$-ATPase alpha3 subunit mRNA expression in rat hippocampus. *Am. J. Physiol.*, **266**, C423–8.

McCabe, J.T. and Bolender, R.P. (1993). Estimation of tissue mRNAs by *in situ* hybridization. *J. Histochem. Cytochem.*, **41**, 1777–83.

Mohammed, A.H., Henriksson, B.G., Soderstrom, S., Ebendal, T., Olsson, T., and

Seckl, J.R. (1993). Environmental influences on the central nervous system and their implications for the aging rat. *Behav. Brain Res.*, **57**, 183–91.

Olsson, T., Mohammed, A.H., Donaldson, L.F., Henriksson, B.R., and Seckl, J.R., (1994). Glucocorticoid receptor and NGFI-A gene expression are induced in the hippocampus after environmental enrichment in adult rats. *Mol. Brain Res.*, **23**, 349–53.

Yau, J.L.W., Kelly, P.A.T., Sharkey, J., and Seckl, J.R. (1994). Chronic 3,4-methylenedioxymethamphetamine (MDMA) administration decreases glucocorticoid and mineralocorticoid receptor, but increases 5-HT$_{1C}$ receptor gene expression in the rat hippocampus. *Neuroscience*, **61**, 31–40.

7

Detection of genetic changes in cancer by interphase cytogenetics and comparative genomic hybridization

ANTON H.N. HOPMAN, CHRISTINA E.M. VOORTER, ERNST
J.M. SPEEL, FRANS C.S. RAMAEKERS, and PETER G. VOOIJS

Introduction

Quantitative and structural aberrations in the genomic content of malignancies or premalignant lesions, are, in many cases, correlated with prognosis of the disease. Since such genetic changes are central to the initiation and progression of neoplasms, techniques have been developed for their detection and characterization.

Cytogenetic, flow cytometric, and molecular genetic studies have provided convincing evidence that the development and progression of human malignancies involves multiple genetic changes. In this respect karyotyping of tumours allows the determination of numerical and/or structural chromosomal defects. However, chromosome analysis of solid cancers using this conventional cytogenetic technique is, in general, only possible after culturing of isolated tumour cells and can only be performed to a limited extent in a routine setting. Moreover, paraffin-embedded material from patients with known clinical outcome, is, so far, not available for such cytogenetic analyses. The DNA index of many tumour types is regarded as a prognostic parameter. Therefore, flow cytometric (FCM) and morphometric analysis of cells isolated from fresh tumours, or nuclei isolated from paraffin blocks, have become established methods for rapid and objective screening of malignant tumours. Although these later techniques allow the estimation of the total DNA content of large cell populations, no precise information about chromosome aberrations can be obtained. Molecular genetic techniques such as Southern blot, restriction fragment length polymorphism (RFLP) analyses, PCR-based microsatellite analysis, or single strand conformational polymorphism (SSCP) analyses provide information about changes in the number of copies of DNA sequences, loss of heterozygosity, or even mutations in the gene. Because of the integral nature of these approaches such studies are limited to the description of the characteristics of tumours as a whole, without providing any further information about the heterogeneity of cells within the tumour.

Fluorescence *in situ* hybridization (FISH or ISH) technique using chromosome-specific probes, allows targeted detection of numerical chromosome aberrations in the interphase nucleus, and is generally refered to as 'interphase cytogenetics' (Cremer *et al.* 1986). Developments in probe-labelling techniques, generation of different types of probes, and technical improvements for the processing of biological material have now reached such a point that FISH can be considered as a significant adjunct to the more established methods for detection and characterization of genetic aberrations in cancer (Fig. 7.1). FISH methods have not only been applied to several types of malignancies but have also been successfully applied to a variety of cell and tissue preparations, such as single cells isolated from solid cancers collected as paraffin-embedded material or as frozen tissue blocks (reviewed by Lichter *et al.* 1991; McNeil *et al.* 1991; Tkachuk *et al.* 1991; Trask 1991; Poddighe *et al.* 1992; Bentz *et al.* 1994; Hopman *et al.* 1994; Joos *et al.* 1994). The FISH technique offers the possibility of correlating genomic changes to cellular

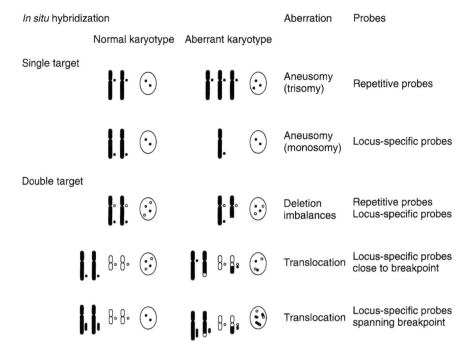

Fig.7.1. Schematic representation of genetic analysis using non-radioactive *in situ* hybridization of metaphase chromosomes and interphase nuclei.

Table 7.1 Detection of genomic aberrations in solid tumours

Technique	Specificity	Histological information	Detection heterogeneity	Detection tetraploid
Karyotyping	High	–	Limited	Limited
Flow cytometry	Low	–	Limited $[G_2M (dipl) = G_0G_1 (tetr)]$	Limited
RFLP	High	–	Mixing normal/aberrant	–
ISH	High	+	+ $[G_2M (dipl) \neq G_0G_1 (tetr)]$	+
CGH	High	–	Mixing normal/aberrant	–

phenotypes on a single cell basis. A correlation with histological features, with proliferative index, or with protein markers has become feasible because of new protocols for application of FISH on sections, or FISH in combination with immunocytochemical approaches.

Recently comparative genomic *in situ* hybridization (CGH) has been developed (Kallioniemi *et al.* 1992; Du Manoir *et al.* 1993). With this technique, based on ISH using isolated tumour DNA as a probe, it is possible to generate a copy number karyotype from, for example, a solid tumour, by comparing the DNA of this tumour with that of normal cells. In contrast with the targeted analysis of FISH, no intact tumour cells are needed nor is the preparation of high quality metaphase spreads from tumour cells required. Furthermore, CGH enables a total mapping of genetic imbalances in the whole tumour genome and is not restricted to the FISH probe or RFLP probe regions only. Table 7.1 summarizes the potential of the different techniques to study genetic changes.

Technical aspects of in situ hybridization

For hybridization and detection protocols, which we apply to single cell suspensions prepared from solid tumours, tumour cell lines, imprints, cytological preparations, and to paraffin and frozen tissue sections of solid tumours, the following general outline can be used.

1. Selection of probes for interphase cytogenetics, probe modification for non-isotopic detection.
2. Fixation of the biological material, slide preparation, and pre-treatments of tissue material on the slides.
3. Hybridization of the modified probe with denatured target DNA, washing, and immunocytochemical detection.
4. Evaluation and interpretation of ISH signals.

DNA probes for interphase cytogenetics

For the detection of numerical and structural chromosome aberrations several different type of probes are available (see Fig. 7.2).

Probes recognizing highly repetitive sequences

DNA probes recognizing repeated DNA sequences in tandem (referred to as *repetitive probes*, *repeat sequence probes*, or *satellite probes*), which are mostly present in the centromeric and telomeric region, are now routinely applicable in daily practice (Willard and Waye 1987; van Dekken *et al.* 1990; Poddighe *et al.* 1992). The sequences targeted by these probes are typically alpha satellite or satellite III sequences that are usually repeated several hundred- to several thousand-fold. This results in DNA targets up to several thousand kilobase pairs (kb) localized in the compact centromeric and telomeric regions of the individual chromosomes. Such repetitive probes have been developed for most of the human chromosomes and many are now commercially available (Oncor, Gaithersburg, Maryland, USA; Imagenetics, Naperville, Illinois, USA; American Type Culture Collection, Rockville, USA; Amersham, Buckinghamshire, UK). The signal intensity of these probes is high and the hybridization signal is tightly localized in metaphase and interphase nuclei. Since the number of signals is constant during the cell cycle these probes can be scored rapidly and accurately.

Fig. 7.2. (a,b) Double target ISH on human metaphase chromosomes and interphase cells with centromere satellite probes for chromosomes 1 (1q13), in red (TRITC), and 18, in green (FITC) (Hopman *et al.* 1988). Counterstaining with DAPI (a). (c) Selectively staining of an entire human X chromosome with a painting probe in a human hamster cell line containing one human X chromosome. (d) Detection of a 40 kb (locus-specific) probe for the chromosome 11q23 region with alkaline phosphatase Fast Red fluorescence in a human lymphocyte metaphase spread, counterstained with thiazole orange (Speel *et al.* 1992). (e,f) Hybridization in bladder tumour cells showing a trisomy for 1q13 (centromere satellite probe) in red (TRITC) (a). Double target ISH for 1q13 and chromosome 18 (centromere satellite probe) in green (FITC). Arrow in e indicates a split spot (counted as one chromosome complement for 1q13). Arrow in f indicates cell with a trisomy for 1q13 and a disomy for chromosome 18. Counterstaining with DAPI (blue) (Hopman *et al.* 1988). (h) Hybridization on a bladder tumour cell line (T24) showing a trisomy for 1q13 and a tetrasomy for 1p36 (centromeric and telomeric satellite probes). Double target hybridization in brown (peroxidase/DAB) and green (peroxidase/TMB) for 1q13 and 1p36, respectively (Speel *et al.* 1994b). Counterstaining haematoxylin. Triple target hybridization in T24 cells with centromeric satellite probes for chromosomes 1, 7 and 17 visualized in brown (peroxidase/DAB), red (alkaline phosphatase/Fast Red, and green (peroxidase/TMB), respectively. No DNA counterstaining (Speel *et al.* 1994b). (j) Combined immunocytochemistry and ISH on a human lung cancer cell. Nuclear detection of Ki67 antigen with alkaline phosphatase/Fast Red (red, fluorescence) in combination with satellite probe for 1q13 (green) (Speel *et al.* 1994a). (k) Immunocytochemical detection of vimentin filaments in blue (β-galactosidase/BCIG) in combination with triple target hybridization on chromosomes 1, 7, and 17 (as seen in i) in a human epithelial cell. No counterstaining (Speel *et al.* 1994b). (See plate section.)

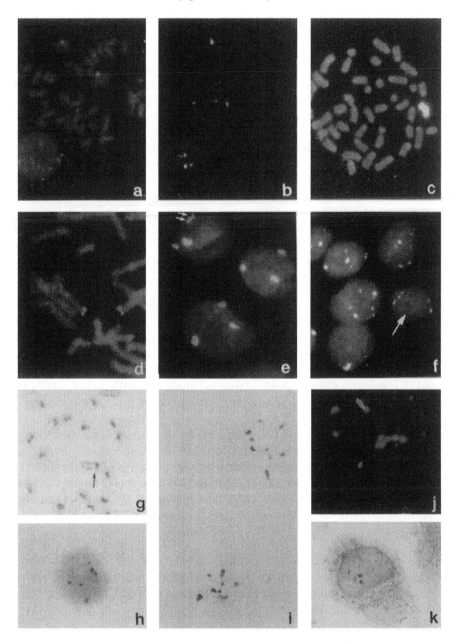

Chromosome painting probes

Another type of DNA probe comprises many different elements distributed densely and more or less continuously over the chromosome so that the probe specifically stains almost the complete chromosome or human chromosome fragment (Cremer *et al.* 1988; Pinkel *et al.* 1988). These so called *whole chromosome probes* or *chromosome painting probes* are based on chromosome purification by fluorescence-activated sorting and subsequent cloning into a vector. Different cloning systems have been developed. Painting probes are now commercially available for several human chromosomes (BRL, Gaithersburg, Maryland, USA; American Type Culture Collection, Rockville, USA; Amersham, Buckinghamshire, UK; Boehringer Mannheim, Mannheim, Germany; CAMBIO, Cambridge, UK). ISH with these probes stains entire chromosomes in metaphase and in interphase nuclei. In the interphase nucleus the FISH domain size is much larger than for the repeat sequence probes. Domain overlap and/or fragmentation hampers chromosome counting in tumours with a complex karyotype.

Locus-specific probes

These probes are useful for analysis of small DNA sequences. They target to unique sequences ranging in size from about 2 kb to a few hundred kb. Different cloning systems, e.g. cosmid, phage, or plasmid vectors and yeast artificial chromosomes (YAC), have been used (Tkachuk *et al.* 1991; Trask 1991; Lichter and Cremer 1992; Matsumar *et al.*, 1992; Ried *et al.* 1992). For chromosome painting probes as well as specific locus probes, suppression of hybridization signals from ubiquitous repeated sequences, such as the *Alu* and *Kpn*1 elements is necessary. This can be achieved by using either total human DNA of *Cot*1 DNA in a reannealing procedure, and is therefore also referred to as chromosome *in situ* suppression hybridization (CISS hybridization). In interphase cytogenetics a high hybridization efficiency is obtained with probes of 30 kb (unique sequences) or larger for analysis of the copy number and structural integrity of several genes (e.g. tumour suppressor genes, oncogenes). In some cases overlapping probes (contig probes) are used to span a large target on the chromosome. Several probes, e.g. for the detection of translocation (*bcr/abl*), or oncogenes (N-*myc*, *HER-2/neu*) are available (Oncor, Gaithersburg, Maryland, USA). Additional probes will be available in the near future as a result of the international human genome project.

Probe modifications

In the last decade about 20 different hapten labelling and fluorochrome labelling procedures have been developed (reviewed by Raap *et al.* 1989). Two major approaches to the labelling or probes can be distinguished: labelling by chemical reaction or labelling mediated by enzymatic polymerization. By chemical modification, large quantities of probe can be modified and the chemical reactions, when well standardized, have high reproducibility. However, for most of the chemical labelling approaches no kits are commercially available. For this reason enzymatic labelling of probes is the method of choice (see Chapter 3). Three of the labels, biotin, digoxigenin, and fluorochrome, are the most frequently used hapten modifications nowadays.

Tumour processing for *in situ* hybridization

Several standard tissue fixatives, such as methanol–acetic acid (3:1) used for karyotyping analyses, 70% ethanol for flow cytometrical analyses, methanol–acetone for cytological analyses, and 4% paraformaldehyde in phosphate buffer saline (PBS) for histopathological analyses, are fully compatible with the *in situ* hybridization procedure. Fresh tumour material obtained after surgery or by thin needle aspiration biopsies can be divided for the different diagnostic approaches (histopathological, immunocytochemical, and cytological). The individual tumour blocks may be treated as follows.

(a) Storage in liquid nitrogen and subsequent cryosectioning.

(b) Fixation in 4% paraformaldehyde, phosphate-buffered saline (PBS) for different time periods, up to 24 hours, and embedding in paraffin. These tissue blocks are used for routine histopathological diagnosis, immunocytochemistry, and ISH on 4–7 µm sections.

(c) Preparation of single cell suspensions for FCM and ISH. In brief, the tissues are mechanically disaggregated by scraping and cutting in a Petri dish and filtered through a 100 µm nylon filter (Ortho Diagnostic Systems, Beerse, Belgium). The filtered cell suspensions are fixed in 70% ethanol ($-20\,°C$) and stored for some months, up to several years, at $-30\,°C$.

Slide preparation and pre-treatment of tissues

In order to detect specific nucleic acid sequences, DNA probes (and antibodies) have to penetrate complex and dense biological structures to reach their targets. For this reason the biological material has to be pre-treatment to increase the accessibility of these DNA targets. During this permeabilization step, however, isolated cells or parts of tissue sections may be lost if they are attached to non-coated glass slides. Slides can be coated with: (a) poly-L-lysine; (b) gelatin–chrome–alum coating; and (c) aminoalkylsilane. If needed, a covalent cross-linking of cellular material is possible after glutaraldehyde activation of these coated slides (see Appendix, Protocol 1).

Single cells

Single cell suspensions can be relatively and easily isolated by mechanical or enzymatic disaggregation of fresh biological material, frozen tissue sections, and paraffin-embedded solid tumours (Hopman *et al.* 1988, 1991, 1992; Emmerich *et al.* 1989a; van Dekken *et al.* 1990, 1992b; Arnoldus *et al.* 1991a; Poddighe *et al.* 1991; Waldman *et al.* 1991). Protocols specified for interphase cytogenetics of solid tumours have been developed. Removal of cytoplasm and nuclear proteins can be achieved by alcohol–acetic acid fixation prior to spotting of the cells on to the pre-treated glass slides, followed by a mild permeabilization step, or by enzymatic digestion after spotting of ethanol-fixed cells. In the latter case the fixation procedure is identical to that used for flow cytometric analyses. Ethanol-fixed cell suspensions can be stored for years without any reduction in ISH ability following Protocol 2 described in the Appendix. To optimize the specificity and intensity of the ISH signal for detection of the correct chromosomal copy number, the pepsin concentration and digestion time need to be optimized or tuned. An underestimation of the chromosome copy number can easily be made when the pepsin concentration is too low, while a large heterogeneity in chromosome copy numbers can be detected as a result of loss of morphology if the cells are overdigested. A standard digestion schedule of 100 µg pepsin/ml in 0.01 M HCl for 20 min could be used for several tumour types, including bladder cancer, renal cell cancer, leukaemia, and several different ethanol-fixed tumour cell lines. If tissue or cell morphology is completely lost as a result of the digestion, evaluation of the signals cannot be done properly, and an additional step of baking the slides, or extra fixation steps, should be included in the protocol to reach an acceptable morphology. The protocol could also be used, for example, for cytological preparation, imprints, or cells isolated from villi for prenatal diagnosis.

Paraffin-embedded tumour material

A number of studies have dealt with the application of ISH to the study of chromosomal aberrations in the cell nucleus of routinely processed, paraffin-embedded tissues (Burns *et al.* 1985; Naoumov *et al.* 1988; Emmerich *et al.* 1989b; Arnoldus *et al.* 1991a; Hopman *et al.* 1991b; van Dekken *et al.* 1992b. Dhingra *et al.* 1994; Thompson *et al.* 1994). We compared the number of ISH signals detected in ethanol-fixed single cell suspensions of a large series of bladder tumours with the ISH results obtained in paraffin sections of the same tumours (Hopman *et al.* 1991b). The correlation between the ISH spot numbers counted for a specific chromosome in the cell suspensions and those counted in the paraffin sections was best in low grade, diploid, transitional cell carcinomas. When aneuploid cancers were studied the spot numbers counted in paraffin gave an underestimation of the real copy number of individual chromosomes, in particular because the aneuploid nuclei were in general larger than the diploid nuclei. As a result truncation of nuclei was a more significant problem in these former tumour types.

The added value of ISH on paraffin sections compared with ISH on isolated tumour cells can be summarized as follows.

(1) The focal tumour cell areas with chromosome aberrations can be recognized in the sections and correlated with histological appearance.

(2) No selection of cells occurs as a result of the isolation procedure.

(3) Heterogeneity, as well as tetraploidization within the tumour can be recognized.

(4) It allows retrospective analysis using archival material.

However, in daily practice this procedure may have its limitations, since, for each paraffin block, the proteolytic pre-treatment step has to be optimized. The success rate of ISH is mainly dictated by the accessibility of the target DNA. Proteolytic enzymes such as pepsin and proteinase K are generally and efficiently used to permeabilize the tissue section to allow penetration of modified probes and antibodies. Additional steps to improve the ISH reaction include: (a) deparaffinization in warm xylol; (b) freezing and thawing of the cells; (c) prolonged digestion time; (d) increased denaturation temperatures; and (e) different treatment steps prior to enzymatic digestion. However, no data concerning reproducibility on large series of paraffin-embedded tumour blocks are available. To improve the efficiency of the ISH procedure using pepsin in 0.2 M HCl for permeabilization of the section, a DNA–nucleohistone denaturation or dissociation step by heating in hot 1 M sodium thiocyanate (80°C) could be included. Pre-treatment of the sections in this way strongly improves the effect of the proteolytic digestion step, resulting in reproducible and efficient ISH results. In Protocol 3 (see Appendix) guidelines for the ISH procedure on paraffin sections, tested on routinely processed malignancies from bladder, mesothelioma, ovarian carcinoma, hydatidiform moles, abortions, and lymphoma are given. As mentioned before, for each tissue block the proteolytic digestion time should be optimized, taking a series of digestion time periods, ranging from 5 min up to 60 min. The sodium thiocyanate treatment is optional and is only suggested when the ISH reaction is negative under standard conditions. Since different cell types (tumour cells, inflammatory cells, stromal cells) may need different optimal pre-treatment conditions, optimization should of course be directed towards the cell type of interest. The standard digestion time for a 4–6 μm section is 30 min at 37°C in 4 mg pepsin per ml 0.2 M HCl, with a denaturation time of 8 min at 80°C. Following this protocol, we obtained good ISH signals in 90% of the tumours examined.

Frozen sections

So far no detailed protocol has been published dealing with the detection of numerical or structural chromosome aberrations in a large series of frozen tissue sections of solid tumours. In general, frozen sections can be mildly fixed in methanol–acetone or, more strongly, in formaldehyde. Proteolytic digestion should be tuned not to overdigest the cells, which results in a complete loss of morphology. Protocol 4 in the Appendix gives a suggestion of how to optimize ISH on frozen sections.

Hybridization of probes and immunocytochemical detection

After hybridization of the probe (in most cases overnight) stringent post-hybridization washings are performed to remove unspecifically hybridized probes. Washings for satellite probes are normally done in 60% formamide, $2 \times$ SSC at 42 °C for 10 minutes; and painting and locus-specific probes in 50% formamide, $2 \times$ SSC at 42 °C also for 10 min (see articles describing the specific probes). After these washings, in most cases, the haptens are detected by standard affinity cytochemical techniques. In the case of biotin, for example, the reporter molecule can be detected with labelled (strept)avidin molecules or monoclonal anti-biotin followed by incubation with labelled second antibodies. Labels can be fluorochromes, like fluorescein (FITC), rhodamine (TRITC), and aminomethyl-coumarin acetic acid (MACA), or enzymes, such as peroxidase and alkaline phosphatase (see Tables 7.2 and 7.3; reviewed by Bentz *et al.* 1994; Raap *et al.* 1992; Speel *et al.* 1994b, 1995). In the case of fluorochrome-labelled DNA probes no immunological detection is needed, although an immunological amplification step to obtain a higher signal intensity using anti-fluorochrome antibodies and second antibodies is possible (Weigant *et al.* 1991). The choice of detection system will depend on the area of application of the *in situ* hybridization and the choice of microscope. In the case of enzymatic detection (visualization by bright-field microscopy) the preparation will be permanent, the detection and evaluation is not influenced by, for example, autofluorescence of the specimen, and different substrates can result in precipitated products of different colours. In the case of fluorescent detection (visualization by fluorescence microscope) a higher detection intensity and sharper localization is obtained (detection limit up to a few kb).

Table 7.2 Detection of labelled probes

Label	Immunochemical detection system/affinity detection system		
	Primary layer	**Secondary layer**	**Third layer**
Biotin	Avidin*		
	Avidin*	Biotinylated anti-avidin	Avidin*
	Mouse anti-biotin*	Rabbit anti-mouse*	
		Biotinylated anti-mouse	Avidin*
Dig	Mouse anti-dig*	Anti-mouse*	
		Biotinylated anti-mouse	Avidin*
		Dig-labelled anti-mouse	Anti-dig*
	Rabbit anti-dig*	anti-rabbit*	
FITC	Rabbit-anti-FITC	Swine anti-rabbit*	
	Mouse-anti-FITC	Anti-mouse*	

Dig: digoxigenin; FITC: fluorescein.
*Proteins can be conjugated with a fluorochrome or enzyme (see Table 7.3).

Table 7.3 Detection of labelled probes

Enzymes/ fluorochromes	Substrate	Detection
Peroxidase	H_2O_2/DAB (brown colour)	Bright-field microscopy
	H_2O_2/chloronaphthol (purple colour)	Bright-field microscopy
	H_2O_2/TMB (green colour)	Bright-field microscopy
Alkaline phosphatase	BCIP/NBT (blue colour)	Bright-field microscopy
	Naphthol-p/Fast Red (red colour)	Bright-field microscopy
	(red fluorescence)	Fluorescence microscopy
	Naphthol-p/New Fuchsin (red colour)	Bright-field microscopy
	(red fluorescence)	Fluorescence microscopy
Fluorochromes	FITC (green, yellow fluorescence)	Flourescence microscopy
	AMCA (blue fluorescence	Flourescence microscopy
	TRITC; CY3 (red fluorescence)	Flourescence microscopy
	TexasRed (red fluorescence)	Flourescence microscopy
	CY5 (infrared fluorescence)	Flourescence microscopy

Evaluation and interpretation of ISH signals
In situ hybridization on single cell suspensions

Fluorescent ISH signals are evaluated by counting, for example, 200 nuclei (Hopman *et al.* 1988, 1991a). It is assumed that the chromosome copy number is identical to the number of hybridization signals obtained with its specific centromeric probe. One should realize that in a mixed normal and tumour cell population the number of interphase nuclei that need to be analysed for a valid evaluation of monosomy or trisomy, for example is dependent on the frequency of the tumour cells in the total cell population. Not only the frequency, but also the percentage of false positive cells is important (for details, see Kibbelaar *et al.* 1993). The percentage of false positive cells has been shown to be strongly dependent on the pre-treatment of the biological material.

The percentage of cells without ISH signal differs from experiment to experiment and percentages of 10% artificial 'nullisomy' are not uncommon. However, with optimal pre-treatment steps (e.g. optimal pepsin treatment, no autofluorescence background covering part of nucleus) this percentage could be reduced to less then 3%. Especially in flow cytometrically determined aneuploid and tetraploid tumours, a high percentage of negative cells (>15% will inevitably lead to an underestimation of the chromosome copy number or tumour heterogeneity. The percentage of nuclei with one ISH signal in diploid cells differs from 5 to 20%, again depending on the efficiency of the ISH procedure. There is always a certain percentage of the nuclei that shows one ISH signal as a result of colocalization of ISH signals. When the number of cells with one signal per nucleus is above 20% of the population, this can be regarded as a strong indication for monosomy of the particular chromosome, although by double-target hybridizations this arbitrary minimum percentage could be reduced to 10%. An indication of trisomy or tetrasomy can be reached at a cell ratio exceeding 5% (arbitrary) of the total cell population. This percentage can also be determined by taking three times the standard deviation aberrant from the mean in a control group (Anastasi *et al.* 1990). Overlapping nuclei, as well as minor hybridization signals and pairing of ISH signals, should not be included in the evaluation. Some typical pitfalls that may occur during the interpretation of chromosome aneuploidy using ISH are summarized as follows.

1. Pairing of chromosomes, resulting in one ISH signal that could be interpretated as a monosomy. For example, in normal brain tissue somatic pairing of chromosomes 1 and 17 (centromere pairing) has been found (Arnoldus *et al.* 1991b), as well as pairing of the short arm of chromosomes 15 in haematopoetic and lymphoid systems (Lewis *et al.* 1993).

2. Translocations of short arm sequences from chromosome 15 on to other D-group chromosomes occur frequently. ISH studies with a chromosome 15-specific probe will then show three ISH signals in the interphase nuclei, suggesting a trisomy for chromosome 15 (Smeets *et al.* 1991).

3. Paired arrangement of ISH signals could indicate: (i) a split spot (for satellite probes) suggesting two copies (Hopman *et al.* 1988), but this should be interpreted as one chromosome complement (this phenomenon has been shown to be cell cycle independent); or (ii) a doublet of ISH spots (for locus-specific probes) indicating a replicated DNA segment that is cell cycle dependent but also should be counted as one chromosome complement (Selig *et al.* 1992).

4. Chromosomal polymorphisms, e.g. in chromosome 1 and 9, resulting in heterogeneity of ISH signal intensities with chromosome-specific satellite DNA sequences. Interpretation of minor specific hybridization signals (still present after stringent washings) as a minor binding site will lead to an underestimation of the chromosome copy number (Hopman *et al.* 1992).

The following criteria should be applied for proper evaluation with minimal interobserver variation (Devilee *et al.* 1988; Hopman *et al.* 1988).

(a) Overlapping nuclei are not counted.

(b) Nuclei are evaluated in which the ISH signals have more or less the same homogeneous fluorescence intensity, unless indications of a partial deletion or polymorphism exist.

(c) Minor hybridization signals, which can be recognized by a lower intensity and spot area, are not counted.

(d) Fluorescent spots or patches of fluorescence in nuclei are included when the signals are completely separated.

In situ hybridization on sections

For the evaluation of ISH signals in paraffin-embedded or frozen tissue sections, the same criteria can be followed as used for single cell suspensions (Fig. 7.3). However, for sections, the percentage of cells with no or one signal for normal ploidy will be higher (about 25%) compared with the single cell suspension (about 5%). In paraffin-embedded and frozen tissue sections the results will be more qualitatively evaluated (selection of tumour area, normal tissue, stromal cells), since no simple correction factors for truncation of nuclei are available. Recently, a statistical approach to analyse monosomies and trisomies has been published and deals more with the quantitative evaluation of the tissue section hybridizations (Dhingra *et al.* 1994). In flow cytometrically determined diploid tumours the size of the nuclei will range from 4 to 6 μm. In these tumours the effect of truncation on the detectability of the real chromosome copy number will be limited. In about 50% of the nuclei the true chromosome copy number should be detectable, so that a monosomy and trisomy can be decided upon. In aneuploid and tetraploid tumours, which range between 6 and 13 μm in nuclear size (depending on DNA content), an evident underestimation of the chromosome copy number will be made as a result of truncation of the nuclei (Hopman *et al.* 1991b). With increasing nuclear size the real chromosome copy number will be even more underestimated. However, an indication of the real chromosome copy number can be obtained by taking the maximum number of ISH signals per nucleus as the chromosome copy number. By hybridization of serial sections (in one experiment using the same section thickness and the same proteolytic pre-treatment), or double-target hybridizations using different chromosomal probes, the imbalance between chromosome copy numbers can be determined. In dense cell areas, the overlap of nuclei complicates the evaluation of signals per individual nucleus, since the morphology is partly disrupted during the hybridization. In these cases a laminin immunocytochemical staining of the nuclear contour facilitates evaluation of the *in situ* hybridization signals (Herbergs personal communication; see Fig. 7.3). The best estimation of the true chromosome copy number could be deduced from ISH results in paraffin sections that were enzymatically treated for different times, resulting in good morphology up to a complete loss of morphology. Prolonged treatment will normally result in an increase in the number of ISH signals by misinterpretation of nuclear shape. Hybridization of thick tissue sections and evaluation of *in situ* hybridization signals by confocal microscopy is another approach; however, for routine application this is rather complicated (Thompson *et al.* 1994). An alternative approach to detect more validly the true chromosome copy number in paraffin, as well as frozen sections, is the isolation of nuclei from thick tissue sections (Arnoldus *et al.* 1991a; Hyytinen *et al.* 1994; van Lijnschoten *et al.* 1994). Truncation of nuclei will be reduced compared with the thin sections used for direct hybridization on sections.

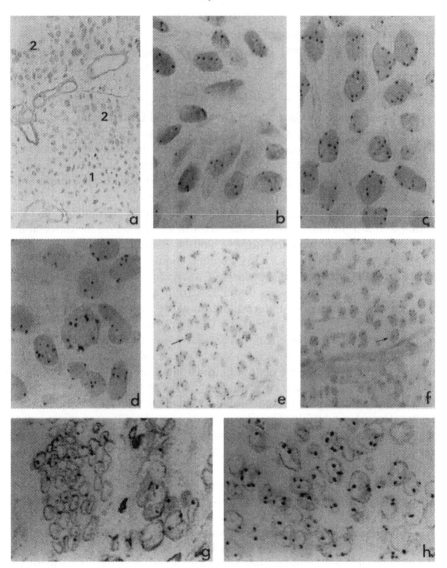

Fig. 7.3. (a–f) Hybridization in paraffin-embedded tissue sections of bladder tumours (a–f, transitional cell carcinomas) and colon cancers (g,f) with centromere satellite probes. Targets for chromosomes 7 (a–d) and 1 (1q13) (e,f), 18 (g), and 7 (h) were detected with peroxidase/DAB. (a–d) Illustration of heterogeneity within one individual case. In (a) low magnification to illustrate two areas (indicated as areas 1 and 2) containing nuclei with a different nuclear morphology and size. The difference is apparently the result of polyploidization or tetraploidization within the tumour (Hopman *et al.* 1991b; Ramaekers *et al.* 1992). (b) Magnification of area 1 [see (a)]. ISH signal copy number ranged from one to four. In many cells four copies can be seen, indicative of a tetrasomy. (c,d) Magnification of area 2 [see (a)]. Illustration of polysomy for chromosome 7, as a result of nuclear

Comparison of ISH with karyotyping, FCM, and RFLP

Table 7.1 summarizes the effect of the different techniques to study genetic changes.

Karyotyping

Chromosome banding techniques play an important role, mainly in the detection of genetic aberrations of haematological malignancies. Since a well-established knowledge of the chromosome aberrations in these malignancies exists, karyotyping can be used in determining their diagnosis and prognosis. Although karyotyping is routinely applicable in leukaemia, karyotyping of solid tumours might be very cumbersome and selection of a fast-growing subpopulation could give unreliable information about the total tumour population. Furthermore, it is not possible to use archival material with this method.

It is important to realize, however, that extrapolation of interphase cytogenetic data towards true chromosomal aberrations is not without pitfalls either, since the signals obtained from these probes often do not reflect complex structural rearrangements. Such structural changes can involve translocations or deletions of p or q arms, or part of these arms, and therefore selective staining of the complete chromosome, or of carefully chosen cosmid probes, is necessary for detection of these changes in interphase cytogenetics. With double-target ISH experiments on interphase nuclei it has been possible to detect translocations, and even cytogenetically non-characterized marker chromosomes could be recognized blindly by co-localization of ISH signals in double-target ISH procedures. With the ISH method it is also feasible to detect low numbers of host cells (e.g. in sex-mismatched bone marrow transplant recipients) or Philadelphia chromosomes (*BCR–ABL* fusion chromosomes) in leukaemia (Arnoldus *et al.* 1990; Tkachuk *et al.* 1991; Bentz *et al.* 1994).

Data from reported conventional cytogenetic studies of solid tumours could be useful for interphase screening in those cases where karyotyping is lacking. As a consequence of heterogeneity, in cases of a diploid modal chromosome number, cells with a 3*n* and 4*n* chromosome count were frequently detected

---

truncation, the number of signals per nucleus ranged from one to more than 12. Many nuclei showed 5 to 7 ISH signals. (e,f) Illustration of a trisomy [indicated by an arrow in (e)] and polyploidization within the tumour, resulting in nuclei with a multiple copy number [indicated by arrow in (f)]. (g,h) Combined ISH with immunocytochemical lamin staining of the nuclear envelope. Prior to ISH, immunocytochemistry was performed with anti-laminin and alkaline phosphatase/Fast Red for nuclear counterstaining. In areas in which the nuclei are very densely packed, immunocytochemical nuclear contourstaining facilitates the analysis of the number of ISH signals per individual nucleus [see (h), tetrasomy for 1q13]. Courtesy of J. Herbergs, University of Limburg, Maastricht, The Netherlands.

by karyotyping and counting of chromosomes in metaphase plates. In these cases the percentage of interphase nuclei with a chromosomal aberration could be very low (Schapers *et al.* 1993). By analysis of tissue sections these aberrant cells could be specifically localized within small areas or randomly distributed between the other tumour cells. Hybridizations on tissue sections can be used to visualize this heterogeneity (see Fig. 7.3).

Flow cytometry

It is important to realize that with flow cytometry the actual DNA content of the cells is measured and this indicates that no difference can be made between a diploid cell in G_2M phase or a tetraploid cell in G_0G_1 phase. The number of ISH signals (also in paired arrangement) for the different probes is constant during the cell cycle stages, including G_0G_1, S, and G_2M (Beck *et al.* 1992). Thus, ISH enables discrimination between a (flow cytometrically identical) G_2M population of a diploid tumour and a G_0G_1 population of a tetraploid tumour. In these two cases, two ISH signals and four ISH signals for each chromosome are detected, respectively.

It is generally accepted that tetraploidization is a crucial step in the progression of many solid tumours, in which random as well as non-random loss of chromosomes could lead to selection and growth of aneuploid cells. From this perspective it is also feasible that different cell populations can be present in such neoplasms, resulting in a heterogeneous tumour cell population. Interphase cytogenetics is a simple method for studying this genetic tumour heterogeneity, with the following possibilities. (a) ISH enables the detection of tetraploidization in tumours in which no aneuploidy could be detected by flow cytometry. (b) ISH is able to detect 'minor' aberrant cell populations within tumours with a diploid DNA content, as well as a minor tumour population that has undergone tetraploidization. In bladder cancer these minor, tetraploid fractions could be detected by a doubling of the FISH spots compared with the major tumour cell population. (c) Double-target ISH procedure can be used to detect the imbalance between chromosomes within these minor tumour cell populations, since the different chromosomes can be detected simultaneously.

RFLP and PCR-based microsatellite analysis

Comparison of tumour DNA and constitutional DNA for polymorphic markers by restriction fragment length polymorphism (RFLP) or microsatellite analysis allows the detection of loss of heterozygosity (LOH) at specific chromosomal loci. LOH at chromosomal regions in tumour tissue may indicate deletions of putative tumour suppressor genes. For example, allelic loss on 17p (p53) was shown to be involved in various human cancers by RFLP analysis. In principle, allelic losses can be detected by fluorescence *in situ* hybridization if the loss occurs by deletion. Indeed, a correlation was found between LOH for 17p (p13.3), as revealed by RFLP, and deletion of 17p loci in breast cancer cells, detected by FISH using cosmid probes (Matsumar *et al.* 1992). However, in these cases LOH could be detected because the major population of nuclei had a deletion as shown by FISH. In cases of heterogeneous populations (e.g. 90% normal cells) or mixed populations of chromosome diploid and aneuploid cells, RFLP analyses are limited, while using ISH minor aberrant populations can still be detected.

Comparative genomic hybridization (CGH) methodology and evaluation

The principle of the CGH procedure is outlined schematically in Fig. 7.4. Genomic test DNA, isolated from a tumour specimen, is labelled with a hapten (e.g. biotin), whereas genomic control DNA, isolated from normal lymphocytes, is labelled with another hapten (digoxigenin). An equimolar mixture of these differently labelled genomic DNA probes is used for chromosomal *in situ* suppression hybridization on normal metaphase spreads. The hybridized test and control DNA sequences are detected by different fluorochromes (e.g. FITC, TRITC). Since test and control DNA sequences compete for the same target chromosomes (sequences), the relative copy number of tumour sequences is directly reflected by the ratio of the FITC:TRITC fluorescence intensities. The fluorescence signal intensities are

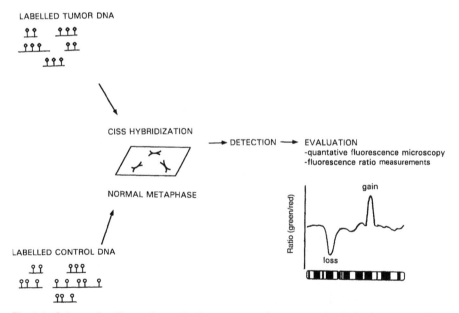

Fig. 7.4. Schematic illustration of the comparative genomic hybridization (CGH). Explanation is given in the text.

measured by quantitative microscopy, using a CCD camera and computer software for imaging and fluorochrome ratio imaging. Karyotyping is done on the basis of DAPI staining of the chromosomes. Amplifications and deletions of 1–10 Mb are detectable, and this sensitivity will be further increased by optimization of the method in the next few years. Concerning the amplifications, even smaller regions of amplification (100 kb) can be detected, if such an amplicon is present in excess (20 times or more). In this respect double-minutes (DMS) or homogeneous staining regions (HSRs) present in the tumour are shown to be amplified sequences as analysed by CGH. Also, imbalances of chromosomes or chromosome arms can be detected with CGH. Compared with other techniques available at present for the evaluation of genetic aberrations of solid tumours, CGH has several major advantages.

1. A complete copy number karyotype can be obtained with this technique, representing truely the isolated tumour DNA. Compared with targeted FISH, the specificity is not limited to the analysis of a specific target gene or chromosome region, but covers the whole genome.

2. Since the technique is based on biochemical isolation of DNA the amount of available tumour material is no longer limiting, because DNA can be amplified by standard PCR technology. In this case the DNA must be amplified by a general DNA amplification method like a degenerate oligonucleotide primed (DOP)-PCR (Telenius *et al.* 1992). As little DNA as that isolated from a few hundred cells is sufficient to obtain proper preparations, after DOP-PCR and nick translation, for CGH analysis.

3. Single cells, frozen tissue blocks or sections, as well a paraffin-embedded tumour tissue samples can be used (Speicher *et al.* 1993). This enables a retrospective study.

4. By isolation of different parts in a tumour, heterogeneity and genomic differences can be studied.

This approach also has its limitations and problems. Balanced chromosome rearrangements and information about the arrangement in a marker chromosome cannot be detected. Furthermore, since only the ratio between fluorescence intensities is measured no information about the ploidy is obtained. For this latter problem targeted FISH analysis to determine the chromosome ploidy can be a solution. To enable CGH analysis, at least 50% of the material should consist of tumour tissue, because mixing with DNA from normal cells will finally mask chromosomal gains and losses. To enrich the fraction of tumour cells from a biopsy, for example, flow cytometric sorting on the basis of DNA content and/or specific immunocytochemical markers can be performed (Beck *et al.* 1992). DNA from these sorted cells can then be isolated and amplified by DOP-PCR.

Applications

The interphase cytogenetic methods described above have been applied to several types of malignancies, including leukaemia, breast cancer, gynaecological tumours, neurological tumours, prostate cancer, testicular tumours, gastric cancer, and urinary bladder cancer. Application of interphase cytogenetics has been extensively reviewed by Lichter *et al.* (1991), McNeil *et al.* (1991), Tkachuk *et al.* (1991), Trask (1991), Poddighe *et al.* (1992), Bentz *et al.* (1994), and Hopman *et al.* (1994). Figure 7.1 gives a simplified scheme of how these genetic aberrations were analysed by using different types of probe in the interphase nucleus. Recent *in situ* hybridizations have compared the results of interphase cytogenetics with conventional cytogenetic analyses of cell lines derived from solid tumours, and in neoplastic cells from bone marrow and peripheral blood. These studies make it clear that *in situ* hybridization is a powerful technique for studying genetic aberrations in total tumour cell populations independently of the growing capacity of the individual tumour cell populations.

A limited number of CGH studies screening solid tumors have been published so far (Speicher *et al.* 1993; Kallioniemi *et al.* 1994; Ried *et al.* 1994), but it is expected that screening of large series of tumours with CGH will indicate as yet unknown tumour-specific chromosomal areas with deletions or amplifications. At that stage targeted ISH analyses can be performed to study the genetic aberrations in more detail. A comparison has already been made between CGH, RFLP, and targeted *in situ* hybridization analyses (Schröck *et al.* 1994; Voorter *et al.* 1995).

Multiple-target *in situ* hybridization

Simultaneous detection of several DNA targets in one and the same nucleus, chromosome spread, or tissue section is possible with probes carrying different haptens, and which are then visualized with different distinguishable affinity systems (Hopman *et al.* 1986; Dauwerse *et al.* 1992; Nederlof *et al.* 1989, 1990; Ried *et al.* 1992; Speel *et al.* 1992; Wiegant *et al.* 1991, 1993). The resolution between two different ISH signals using different fluorochromes, e.g. fluorescein (FITC, yellow-green) in combination with rhodamine (TRITC or Texas Red, red) or coumarin (AMCA, blue), is excellent. For example, in the case of chronic myeloid leukaemia (CML) the reciprocal translocation responsible for this type of leukaemic is characterized by the fusion of the *bcr* gene on chromosome 22 and the *abl* oncogene on chromosome 9. By red labelling at the *bcr* locus and yellow-green labelling at the *abl* locus, the so-called Philadelphia chromosome is visualized in the interphase nucleus by a co-localization of red and yellow-green (Arnoldus *et al.* 1990; Tkachuk *et al.* 1991). Similar approaches have been used to analyse other translocations. Multi-target FISH with multiple-colour probes now enables the detection of

2–12 different probes in one cell based on combination of the three fluorescent colours mentioned.

For bright-field microscopical evaluation, detection of probes is performed by using different enzymes and colour-producing substrates (see Table 7.3). Double-enzymatic detection is mostly based on peroxidase and alkaline phosphatase (Hopman *et al.* 1986; Emmerich *et al.* 1989b; Kerstens *et al.* 1994, Speel *et al.* 1994b), while a triple-enzymatic detection can be performed by combining, for example, two peroxidase and one alkaline phosphatase reaction (see Fig. 7.2; Speel *et al.* 1994b).

Multiparameter analysis

The FISH technique offers the possibility of correlating genomic changes to cellular phenotypes on a single cell basis (van den Brink *et al* 1990; Losada *et al.* 1991; van den Berg *et al.* 1991' Dirks *et al.* 1993; Strehl and Ambros 1993; Weber-Matthiesen *et al.* 1993) Herbergs *et al.* 1994; Speel *et al.* 1994a, 1995). Recently, the application of alkaline phosphatase (APase) Fast Red reaction for the immunocytochemical (ICC) detection of proteins before the ISH step has been reported (Speel *et al.* 1994a). This detection method produces a strongly red fluorescent, permanent reaction product that is resistant to ISH pre-treatments (enzymatic) and procedures. The accurate detection of these parameters in the same cell makes this procedure extremely suitable for detection of tumour cell heterogeneity, rare event detection, and in cases where only a few cell can be obtained for analysis (e.g. in aspirate cytology or in biopsy material). Furthermore, in cases where extensive proteolytic digestion for fluorescence ISH is needed (e.g. in paraffin sections), ICC based on APase/Fast Red can be advantageous. Using this approach cellular markers such as neural cell adhesion molecules, cytokeratin filaments, laminin, or the Ki67 antigen can be combined with ISH using centromere-specific DNA probes.

Acknowledgements

We would like to thank M. Vallinga and Dr P. Poddighe for technical assistance and discussions. We thank Dr J. Herberts (Dept Pathology, University of Limburg, Maastricht, The Netherlands) for kindly providing illustrations for the combined laminin ICC and ISH.

References

Anastasi, J., Le Bau, M.M., Vardiman, J.W., and Westbrook, C.A. (1990). Detection of numerical chromosomal abnormalities in neoplastic hematopoetic cells using *in situ* hybridization with a chromosome specific probe. *Am. J. Pathol.*, **136**, 131–9.

Arnoldus, E.P.J., Wiegant, J., Noordermeer, I.A., Wessels, J.W., Beverstock, C.C.,

Grosveld, G.C., van der Ploeg, M., and Raap, A.K. (1990). Detection of the Philadelphia chromosome in interphase nuclei. *Cytogenet. Cell Genet.*, **54**, 108–11.

Arnoldus, E.P.J., Dreef, E.J., Noordermeer, I.A., Verheggen, M.M., Thierry, R.P., Peters, A.C., Cornelisse, C.J., van der Ploeg, M., and Raap, A.K. (1991a). Feasibility of *in situ* hybridization with chromosome specific DNA probes on paraffin embedded tissue. *J. Clin. Pathol.*, **44**, 900–4.

Arnoldus, E.P.J., Noordermeer, I.A., Peters, A.C.B., Voormolen, J.H.C., Bots, G.T.A.M., Raap, A.K., and van der Ploeg, M. (1991b). Interphase cytogenetics of brain tumours. *Genes Chromosomes Cancer*, **3**, 101–7.

Beck, J.L.M., Hopman, A.H.N., Vooijs, G.P., and Ramaekers, F.C.S. (1992). Chromosome detection by *in situ* hybridization in cancer cell populations which were flow cytometrically sorted after immunolabeling. *Cytometry*, **13**, 346–55.

Bentz, M., Döhner, H., Cabot, G., and Lichter, P. (1994). Fluorescence *in situ* hybridization in leukemias: 'the FISH are spawning'. *Leukemia*, **8**, 1447–52.

Burns, J., Chan, V.T.W., Jonasson, J.H., Fleming, K.A., Taylor, S., and McGee, J.O'D. (1985). Sensitive system for visualizing biotinylated DNA probes hybridized *in situ*: rapid sex determination of intact cells. *J. Clin. Pathol.*, **38**, 1085–92.

Cremer, T., Landegent, J., Bruckner, A., Scholl, H.P., Schardin, M., Hager, H.D., Devilee, P., Pearson, P., and van der Ploeg, M. (1986). Detection of chromosome aberrations in the human interphase nucleus by visualization of specific target DNAs with radioactive and non-radioactive *in situ* hybridization techniques diagnosis of trisomy 18 with probe L1.84. *Hum. Genet.*, **74**, 346–52.

Cremer, T., Lichter, P., Borden, J., Ward, D.C., and Manuelidis, L. (1988). Detection of chromosome aberrations in metaphase and interphase tumor cells by *in situ* hybridization using chromosome-specific library probes. *Hum. Genet.*, **80**, 235–46.

Dauwerse, J.G., Wiegant, J., Raap, A.K., Breuning, M.H., and van Ommen, G.J.B. (1992). Multiple colors by fluorescence *in situ* hybridization using ratio-labelled DNA probes create a molecular karyotype. *Hum. Mol. Genet.*, **1**, 593–8.

Devilee, P., Thierry, R.F., Kievits, T., Kolluri, R., Hopman, A.H.N., Willard, H.F., Pearson, P.L., and Cornelisse, C.J. (1988). Detection of chromosome aneuploidy in interphase nuclei from human primary breast tumors using chromosome-specific repetitive DNA probes. *Cancer Res.*, **48**, 5825–30.

Dhingra, K., Sneige, N., Pandita, T.K., Johnston, D.A., Lee, J.S., Emami, E., Hortobagyi, G.N., and Hittelman, W.N. (1994). Quantitative analysis of chromosome *in situ* hybridization signal in paraffin-embedded tissue sections. *Cytmetry*, **16**, 100–12.

Dirks, R.W., Van de Rijke, F.M., Fujishita, S., van der Ploeg, M., and Raap, A.K. (1993). Methodologies for specific intron and extron RNA localization in cultured cells by haptenized and fluorochromized probes. *J. Cell Sc.*, **104**, 1187–97.

Du Manoir, S., Speicher, M.R., Joos, S., Schröck, E., Popp, S., Döhner, H., Kovacs, G., Robert-Nicoud, M., Lichter, P., and Cremer, T. (1993). Detection of complete and partial chromosome gains and losses by comparative genomic *in situ* hybridization. *Hum. Genet.*, **90**, 590–610.

Emmerich, P., Jauch, A., Hofmann, M-C., Cremer, T., and Walt, H. (1989a). Interphase cytogenetics in paraffin embedded sections from human testicular germ cell tumor xenografts and in corresponding cultured cells. *Lab. Invest.*, **61**, 235–42.

Emmerich, P., Loos, P., Jauch, A., Hopman, A.H.N., Wiegant, J., Higgins, M.J., White, B.N., van der Ploeg, M., Cremer, C., and Cremer, T. (1989b). Double *in situ* hybridization in combination with digital image analysis: a new approach to study interphase chromosome topography. *Exp. Cell Res.*, **181**, 126–40.

Herbergs, J., de Bruïne, A.P., Marx, P.T.J., Vallinga, M.I.A., Stockbrügger, R.W., Ramaekers, F.C.S., and Hopman, A.H.N. (1994). Chromosome aberrations in adenomas of the colon. Proof of trisomy in tumor cells by combined interphase cytogenetics and immunocytochemistry. *Int. J. Cancer*, **57**, 781–5.

Hopman, A.H.N., Wiegant, J., Raap, A.K., Landegent, J.E., van der Ploeg, M., and van Duijn, P. (1986). Bi-color detection of two target DNAs by non-radioactive *in situ* hybridization. *Histochemistry*, **85**, 1–4.

Hopman, A.H.N., Ramaekers, F.C.S., Raap, A.K., Beck, J.L.M., Devilee, P., Van der Ploeg, M., and Vooijs, G.P. (1988). *In situ* hybridization as a tool to study numerical chromosome aberrations in solid bladder tumors. *Histochemistry*, **89**, 307–16.

Hopman, A.H.N., Moesker, O., Smeets, W.G.B., Pauwels, R.P.E., Vooijs, G.P., and Ramaekers, F.C.S. (1991a). Numerical chromosome 1.7.9. and 11 aberrations in bladder cancer detected by *in situ* hybridization. *Cancer Res.*, **51**, 644–51.

Hopman, A.H.N., van Hooren, E., van de Kaa, C.A., Vooijs, G.P., and Ramaekers, F.C.S. (1991b). Detection of numerical chromosome aberrations using *in situ* hybridization in paraffin sections of routinely processed bladder cancers. *Mod. Pathol.*, **4**, 503–13.

Hopman, A.H.N., Poddighe, P., Moesker, O., and Ramaekers, F.C.S. (1992). Interphase cytogenetics: an approach to the detection of genetic aberrations in tumours. In: *Diagnositic molecular pathology. A practical approach*, (ed. K,O'D. McGee and C.S. Herrington), pp. 142–67. Oxford University Press, Oxford.

Hopman, A.H.N., Voorter, C.E.M., and Ramaekers, F.C.S. (1994). Detection of genomic changes in cancer by *in situ* hybridization. *Mol. Biol. Rep.*, **19**, 31–44.

Hyytinen, E., Visakorpi, T., Kallioniemi, A., Kallioniemi, O-P., and Isola, J.J. (1994). Improved technique for analysis of formalin-fixed, paraffin-embedded tumors by fluorescence *in situ* hybridization. *Cytometry*, **16**, 93–9.

Joos, S., Fink, T.M., Rätsch, A., and Lichter, P. (1994). Mapping and chromosome analysis: the potential of fluorescence *in situ* hybridization. *J. Biotechnol.*, **35**, 135–53.

Kallioniemi, A., Kallioniemi, O-P., Sudar, D., Rutovitz, D., Gray, J.W., Waldman, F., and Pinkel, D. (1992). Comparative genomic hybridization for molecular cytogenetic analysis of solid tumors. *Science*, **258**, 818–21.

Kallioniemi, A., Kallioniemi, O-P., Piper, J., Tanner, M., Stokke, T., Chen, L., Smith, H.S., Pinkel, D., Gray, J., and Waldman, F.M. (1994). Detection and mapping of amplified DNA sequences in breast cancer by comparative genomic hybridization. *Proc. Natl. Acad. Sci. USA*, **91**, 2156–60.

Kerstens, H.M.J., Poddighe, P.J., and Hanselaar, A.G.J.M. (1994). Double-target *in situ* hybridization in brightfield microscopy. *J. Histochem. Cytochem.*, **42**, 1071–7.

Kibbelaar, R.E., Kok, F., Dreef, E.J., Kleiverda, J.K., Cornelisse, C.J., Raap, A.K., and Kluin, Ph.M (1993). Statistical methods in interphase cytogenetics: an experimental approach. *Cytometry*, **14**, 716–24.

Lewis, J.P., Tanke, H.J., Raap, A.K., Beverstock, G.C., and Kluin-Nelemans, H.C. (1993). Somatic pairing of centromeres and short arms of chromosomes 15 in the hematopoietic and lymphoid system. *Hum. Genet.*, **92**, 577–82.

Lichter, P. and Cremer, T. (1992). Chromosome analysis by non-isotopic *in situ* hybridization. In: *Human cytogenetics. A practical approach*, pp. 157–92. Oxford University Press, Oxford.

Lichter, P., Boyle, A.L., Cremer, C., and Ward, D.C. (1991). Analysis of genes and chromosomes by non-isotopic *in situ* hybridization. *Genet. Anal. Technol. Appl.*, **8**, 24–35.

Losada, A.P., Wessman, M., Tiainen, M., Hopman, A.H.N., Willard, H.F., Solé, F., Caballín, M., Woessner, S., and Knuutila, S. (1991). Trisomy 12 in chronic lymphocytic leukemia: an interphase cytogenetic study. *Blood*, **78**, 775–83.

Matsumar, K., Kallioniemi, A., Kallioniemi, O., Chern, L., Smith, H.S., Pinkel, D., Gray, J., and Waldman, F.M. (1992). Deletion of chromosome 17p loci in breast cancer cells detected by fluorescence *in situ* hybridization. *Cancer Res.*, **52**, 3474–7.

McNeil, J.A., Villnave Johnson, C., Carter, K.C., Singer, R.H., and Lawrence, J.B. (1991). Localizing DNA and RNA within nuclei and chromosomes by fluorescence *in situ* hybridization. *Genet. Anal. Technol. Appl.*, **8**, 41–58.

Naoumov, N.V., Alexander, G.J.M., Eddleston, A.L.W.F., and Williams, R. (1988). *In situ* hybridisation in formalin fixed, paraffin wax embedded liver specimens: method for detecting human and viral DNA using biotinylated probes. *J. Clin. Pathol.*, **41**, 793–8.

Nederlof, P.M., Robinson, D., Abuknesha, R. Wiegant, J., Hopman, A.H.N., Tanke, H.J., and Raap, A.K. (1989). Three-color-fluorescence *in situ* hybridization for the simultaneous detection of multiple nucleic acid sequences. *Cytometry*, **10**, 20–8.

Nederlof, P.M., van der Flier, S., Wiegant, J., Raap, A.K., Tanke, H.J., Pleom, J.S., and van der Ploeg, M. (1990). Multiple fluorescence *in situ* hybridization. *Cytometry,* **11**, 126–31.

Pinkel, D., Landegent, J., Collins, C., Fuscoe, J., Segraves, R., Lucas, J., and Gray J. (1988). Fluorescence *in situ* hybridization with human chromosome-specific libraries: detection of trisomy 21 and translations of chromosome 4. *Proc. Natl. Acad. Sci. USA*, **85**, 9138–42.

Poddighe, P.J., Moesker, O., Smeets, D., Awwad, B.H., Ramaekers, F.C.S., and Hopman, A.H.N. (1991). Interphase cytogenetics of hematological cancer: comparison of classical karyotyping and *in situ* hybridization using a panel of eleven chromosome specific probes. *Cancer Res.*, **51**, 1959–67.

Poddighe, P.J., Ramaekers, F.C.S., and Hopman, A.H.N. (1992). Interphase cytogenetics of tumors. *J. Pathol.*, **166**, 215–24.

Raap, A.K., Marijnen, J.G.J., Vrolijk, J., and van der Ploeg, M. (1986). Denaturation, renaturation, and loss of DNA during *in situ* hybridization procedures. *Cytometry*, **7**, 235–42.

Raap, A.K., Hopman, A.H.N., and van der Ploeg, M. (1989). Hapten labeling of nucleic acid probe for DNA *in situ* hybridization. In: *Techniques in immunocytochemistry*, (ed. G.R. Bullock and P. Ptrusz), Vol. 4, pp. 167–98.

Raap, A.K., Wiegant, J., and Lichter, P. (1992). Multiple fluorescence *in situ* hybridization for molecular cytogenetics. In *Techniques and methods in molecular biology: non-radioactive labeling and detection of biomolecules*, pp. 343–54. Springer-Verlag, Berlin.

Ramaekers, F., Hopman, A., and Vooijs, P. (1992). Advances in the detection of ploidy differences in cancer by *in situ* hybridization. *Anal. Cel. Pathol.*, **4**, 337–44.

Ried, T., Baldini, A., Rand, T.C., and Ward, D.C. (1992). Simultaneous visualization of seven different DNA probes by *in situ* hybridization using combinatorial fluorescence and digital imaging microscopy. *Proc. Natl. Acad. Sci. USA*, **89**, 1388–92.

Ried, T., Peterson, I., Holtgreve-Gretz, H., Speicher, M., Schröck, E., du Manoir, S., and Cremer, T. (1994). Mapping of multiple DNA gaines and losses in primary small cell lung carcinomas by comparative genomic hybridization. *Cancer Res.*, **54**, 1801–6.

Schapers, R., Smeets, W., Hopman, A., Pauwels, R., Geraedts, J., and Ramaekers, F. (1993). Heterogeneity in bladder cancer as detected by conventional chromosome analysis and interphase cytogenetics. *Cancer Genet. Cytogenet.*, **70**, 56–61.

Schröck, E., Thiel, G., Lozanova, T., du Manoir, S., Meffert, M-C., Jauch, A., Speicher, M.R., Nürnberg, P., Vogel, S., Jänisch, W., Donis-Keller, H., Ried, T., Witkowski, R., and Cremer, T. (1994). Comparative genomic hybridization of human malignant gliomas reveals multiple amplification sites and nonrandom chromosomal gains and losses. *Am. J. Pathol.*, **144**, 1203–18.

Selig, S., Okumura, K., Ward, D.C., and Cedar, H. (1992). Denelineation of DNA replication time zones by fluorescence *in situ* hybridization. *EMBO J.*, **11**, 1217–25.

Smeets, D.F.C.M., Merkx, G.F.M., and Hopman, A.H.N. (1991). Frequent occurrence of translocations of the short arm of chromosome 15 to other D-group chromosomes. *Hum. Genet.*, **87**, 45–8.

Speel, E.J.M., and Schutte, B., Wiegant, J., Ramaekers, F.C.S., and Hopman, A.H.N. (1992). A novel fluorescence detection method for *in situ* hybridization, based on the alkaline phosphatase-fast red reaction. *J. Histochem. Cytochem.*, **40**, 1299–1308.

Speel, E.J.M., Herbergs, J., Ramaekers, F.C.S., and Hopman, A.H.N. (1994a). Combined immunocytochemistry and fluorescence *in situ* hybridization for simultaneous tricolor detection of cell cycle, genomic, and phenotypic parameters of tumor cells. *J. Histochem. Cytochem.*, **42**, 961–6.

Speel, E.J.M., Jansen, M.P.H.M., Ramaekers, F.C.S., and Hopman, A.H.N. (1994b). A novel triple-color detection procedure for brightfield microscopy combining *in situ* hybridization with immunocytochemistry. *J. Histochem. Cytochem.*, **42**, 1299–1307.

Speel, E.J.M., Ramaekers, F.C.S., and Hopman, A.H.N. (1995). Cytochemical detection systems for *in situ* hybridization, and the combination with immunocytochemistry. *Histochem. J.*, **27**, 833–58.

Speicher, M.R., du Manoir, S., Schröck, E., Holtgreve-Grez, H., Scoell, B., Lengauer, C., Cremer, T., and Ried T. (1993). Molecular cytogenetic analysis of formalin fized, paraffin embedded solid tumors by comparative genomic hybridization after universal DNA-amplification. *Hum. Mol. Genet.*, **2**, 1907–14.

Strehl, S. and Ambros, P.F. (1993). Fluorescence *in situ* hybridization combined with immunohistochemistry for highly sensitive detection of chromosome 1 aberrations in neuroblastoma. *Cytogenet, Cell Genet.* **63**, 24–31.

Telenius, H., Pelmear, A.H., Tunnacliffe, A., Carter, N.P., Behmel, A., Ferguson-Smith, M.A., Nordenskjöld, M., Pfragner, R., and Ponder, B.A.J.P. (1992). Cytogenetic analysis by chromosome painting using DOP-PCR amplified flow-sorted chromosomes. *Genes Chromosomes Cancer*, **4**, 257–63.

Thompson, C.T., LeBoit, P.E., Nederlof, P.M., and Gray, J.W. (1994). Thick-section fluorescence *in situ* hybridization on formalin-fixed, paraffin-embedded archival tissue provides a histogenetic profile. *Am. J. Pathol.*, **144**, 237–43.

Tkachuk, D.C., Pinkel, D., Kuo, W-L., Weier, H-U., and Gray, J. (1991). Clinical applications of fluorescence *in situ* hybridization. *Genet. Anal. Technol. Appl.*, **8**, 67–74.

Trask, B. (1991). Fluorescence *in situ* hybridization: applications in cytogenetics and gene mapping. *Trends Genet.*, **7**, 149–54.

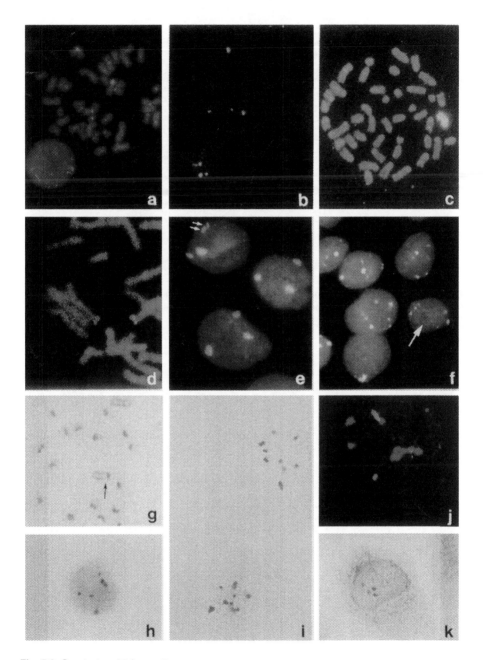

Fig. 7.2: See text, p. 96 for caption.

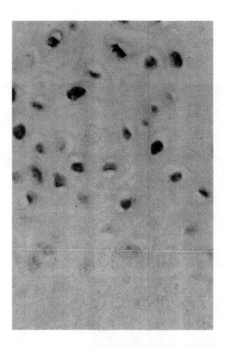

Fig. 8.3: A section from a formalin-fixed, paraffin-embedded condyloma acuminatum was hybridized with an HPV 6 probe. Clear nuclear signal can be seen. (see p. 132)

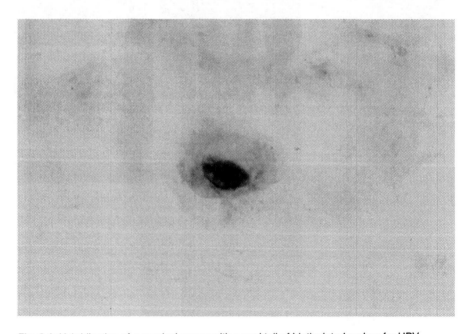

Fig. 8.4: Hybridization of a cervical smear with a cocktail of biotinylated probes for HPV 6,11,16,18,31,33,35. Clear nuclear signal can be seen in both nuclei of a binucleate koilocyte. (see p. 133)

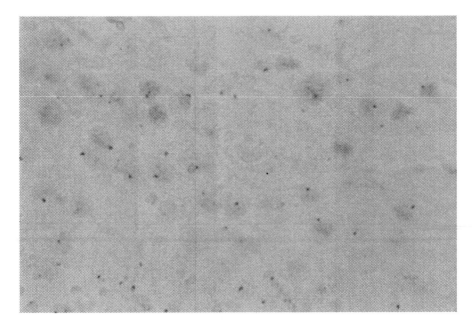

Fig. 8.5: Dual nucleic acid detection: biotinylated HPV 6 probe and digoxigenin-labelled Y chromosome-specific probe were hybridized to a section from a male condyloma acuminatum. The HPV signal can be seen as red and the Y signal as blue dots. (see p. 136)

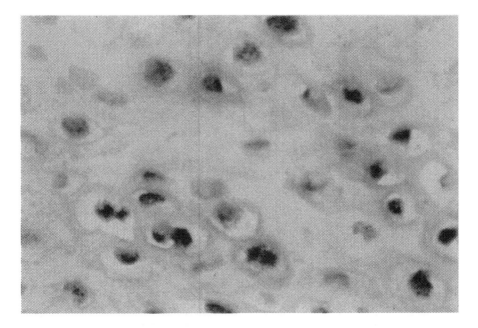

Fig. 8.6: Dual HPV detection: biotinylated HPV 6 and digoxigenin HPV 11 probes were hybridized to a section from a condyloma acuminatum under conditions of low stringency and detected to produce colours as for Fig. 8.5. The signal from both probes can be seen within the same nucleus. (see p. 136)

(a)

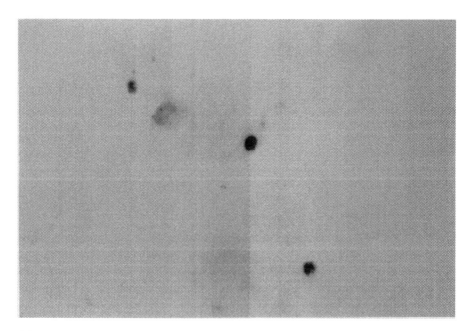

(b)

Fig. 8.8: The application of the dual detection system to cervical smears produces a red signal (a) indicative of HPV 6/11 infection and a blue signal (b) indicative of HPV 16/18/31/33/35 infection. (see p. 138)

van Dekken, H., Pinkel, D., Mullikan, J., and Gray, J. (1988). Enzymatic production of single-stranded DNA as a target for fluorescence *in situ* hybridization. *Chromosoma*, **97**, 1–5.

van Dekken, H., Pizzolo, J.G., Reuter, V.E., and Melamed, M.R. (1990). Cytogenetic analysis of human solid tumors by *in situ* hybridization with a set of 12 chromosome-specific DNA probes. *Cytogenet. Cell Genet.*, **54**, 103–7.

van Dekken, H., Kerstens, H.M., Tersteeg, T.A., Verhofstad, A.A., and Vooijs, G.P. (1992a). Histological preservation after *in situ* hybridization to archival solid tumor sections allows discrimination of cells bearing numerical chromosome changes. *J. Pathol.*, **168**, 317–24.

van Dekken, H., Bosman, F.T., Teijgeman, R., Visssers, G.J., Tersteeg, T.A., Kerstens, H.M., Vooijs, G.R., and Verhofstad, A.A. (1992b). Identification of numerical chromosome aberrations in archival tumours by *in situ* hybridization to routine paraffin sections evaluation of 23 phaeochromocytomas. *J. Pathol.*, **171**, 161–71.

van den Berg, H., Vossen, J.M., Langlois van den Bergh, R., Bayer, J., and van Tol, M.J. (1991). Detection of Y chromosome by *in situ* hybridization in combination with membrane antigens by two-color immunofluorescence. *Lab. Invest.*, **64**, 623–8.

van den Brink, H., van der Loos, C., Volkers, H., Lauwen, H., van den Berg, F., Houthoff, H., and Das, P.K. (1990). Combined β-galactosidase and immunogold/silver staining for immunohistochemistry and DNA *in situ* hybridization. *J. Histochem. Cytochem.*, **38**, 325–9.

van Lijnschoten, G., Albrechts, J., Vallinga, M., Hopman, A.H.N., Arends, J.W., and Geraedts, J.P.M. (1994). Fluorescence *in situ* hybridization on paraffin-embedded abortion material as a means of retrospective chromosome analysis. *Human. Genet.*, **94**, 518–22.

Voorter, C., Joos, S., Brinquier, P-P., Vallinga, M., Poddighe, P., Schalken, J., du Manoir, S., Ramaekers, F., Lichter, P., and Hopman, A. (1995). Detection of chromosomal imbalances in transitional cell carcinoma of the bladder by comparative genomic hybridization. *Am. J. Pathol.*, **146**, 1341–54.

Waldman, F.M., Carroll, P.R., Kerschmann, R., Cohen, M.B., Field, F.G., and Mayall, B.H. (1991). Centromeric copy number of chromosome 7 is strongly correlated with tumor grade and labeling index in human bladder cancer. *Cancer res.*, **14**, 3807–13.

Wang, N., Yi Pan, Heiden, T., and Tribukait, B. (1993). Improved method for release of cell nuclei from paraffin-embedded cell material of squamous cell carcinomas. *Cytometry*, **14**, 931–5.

Weber-Matthiesen, K., Deerberg, J., Müller-Hermelink, A., Schlegelberger, B., and Grote, W. (1993). Rapid immunophenotypic characterization of chromosomally aberrant cells by the new fiction method. *Cytogenet. Cell Genet.*, **63**, 123–5.

Wigant, J., Ried, T., Nederlof, P., van dr Ploeg, M., Tanke, H.J., and Raap, A.K. (1991). *In situ* hybridization with fluoresceinated DNA. *Nucl. Acids Res.*, **19**, 3237–41.

Wiegant, J., Weismeijer, C.C., Hoovers, J.M.N., Schuuring, E., d'Azzo, A., Vrolijk, J., Tanke, H.J., and Raap, A.K. (1993). Multiple and sensitive fluorescence *in situ* hybridization with rhodamine-, fluorescein-, and coumarin-labeled DNAs. *Cytogenet. Cell Genet.* **63**, 73–6.

Willard, F.W. and Waye, J.S. (1987). Hierarchical order in chromosome-specific human alpha satellite DNA. *Trends Genet.*, **3**, 192–8.

Appendix 7.1

Protocol 1. Coating of slides

Method

Glass slides are cleaned in a detergent, e.g. 10% solution of Extran MAO1 (Merck) in distilled water at 60°C for 2 h, rinsed with hot (60°C) tap water, and distilled water, and dried at 80°C.

(a) Poly-L-lysine-coated slides. The slides are dipped for about 20 sec in 1 mg/ml poly-L-lysine (MW >150 000) at room temperature and air-dried (overnight). Coated slides are stores at 4°C.

(b) Alternatively, a gelatin–chrome–alum (GCA) coating may be used. Cleaned slides are incubated in GCA solution (0.5% w/v), gelatin is dissolved in hot water, and, after cooling down to room temperature, 0.05% (w/v) chrome-alum is added at 40°C and air-dried.

(c) Organosilane-coated slides. the slides are incubated overnight in a 2% solution of 3-aminopropyltriethoxysilane in dry acetone. Thereafter, the slides are rinsed in acetone, distilled water (×2), and stored in 0.02% NaN_3 in distilled water. Immediately before use, the slides were rinsed in distilled water and air dried.

Comment. For covalent coupling of cellular material to the glass these slides where chemically activated. Coated slides were activated by immersing them for 15–60 min in 2.5% glutaraldehyde solution in PBS at room temperature in a copling jar. After rinsing the slides with PBS and distilled water they were air-dried. Activation with glytaraldehyde should be done fairly shortly (a few days) before use.

Protocol 2. ISH on single cells (tumour cell lines and isolated cells

Method

Preparation of single cell suspensions for ISH

- Fresh tissues were mechanically disaggregated by scraping and cutting in a Petri dish and filtered through a 100 μm nylon filter.

- After deparaffinization of a 30–50 μm tissue section (paraffin-embedded tissue) nuclei can be isolated by enzymatic disaggregation of the tissue (Wang *et al.* 1993; Hyytinen *et al.* 1994) or mechanical disaggregation of the tissue. After isolation nuclei or cells are further processed (in a tube) following Protocol 3, steps 9–11. Cells are cytospuned or dropped on to the slide.

- Nuclei can be isolated from fresh frozen tissue sections (30–50 μm) by a enzymatic digestion in 100 μg pepsin/ml 0.01 M HCl for 10–20 min at 37 °C.

Fixation and storage

The filtered cell suspensions or tumour cell lines were fixed in 70% ethanol (−20°C) and can be stored for some months up to several years at −20 to −30°C for efficient ISH analysis.

Comment. Alternatively, single tumour cell suspensions can be fixed at 4°C in methanol–acetic acid (3:1) or ethanol–acetic acid (3:1) and stored at −20°C. Shortly before use cells were fixed in freshly prepared methanol–acetic acid (3:1; ×4, 5 min each at 0°C). Two or three drops of the cell suspension were placed on to the coated slides and air -dried. As an option, the remaining cytoplasm was removed or the cells permeabilized by dipping the slides in 70% acetic acid for 10–60 sec or by immersing in 0.1 M HCl, 0.05 Triton X-100 or Tween-20 for 15 min.

ISH method

1. Prepare a cell suspension at approximately 5×10^5 cells/ml and aliquot 5–10 μl on to the slide.

   Comment. The concentration of the cells will vary with the size of the specimen and the aliquot with the cell density required on the slide. If this is desirable, a few cells can be dropped on to the slides, for example, in the case of cytological preparations.

2. Air dry at room temperature for 15 min.

   Comment. If required, for an adequate adhesion of cells, slides are baked for 30–60 min at 80°C.

3. Incubate slides for 20 min at 37°C in 50–400 μg pepsin (porcine stomach mucosa 2500–3500 units per mg protein) per ml 0.01 M HCl. Optimum conditions should be determined.

   Comment. 100 μg/ml is standard. For a mild permeabilization slides can be immersed in 0.1 M HCl, 0.05 Triton X-100, or Tween-20 for 15 min.

4. Rinse slides in H_2O (5 × dip washes) and PBS (5 × dip washes).

5. Post-fixation of cells in 1% formaldehyde in PBS for 10 min at room temperature.

6. After fixation, slides are rinsed in PBS (5 × dip washes).

7. Slides are dehydrated in 70, 90, and 100% ethanol (3 min each) and air-dried.

   Comments. After fixation slides can also be rinsed in 2 × SSC prior to application of the probe under a coverslip; if required, for an adequate adhesion of cells, slides are baked for 30–60 min at 80°C.

8. Apply the probe (1–3 ng/μl) in hybridization buffer (5–10 μl) under a coverslip. Seal the coverslip with rubber cement (not mandatory).

9. Denature slides at 70–60 °C for 2–4 min.

   Comments. 3 min at 70 °C is standard; probe and target DNA can be denaturated separately. Target DNA is denaturated by immersing the slides in 70% formamide, 2 × SSC for 3 min, slides are dehydrated in an ethanol series (4 °C). Different denaturation protocols have been described before (Raap *et al.* 1986; van Dekken *et al.* 1988)

10. Hybridize in a moist chamber overnight at 37 °C.

    Comment. For the centromere-repetitive (satellite) probes a 2 h hybridization step is sufficient.

Protocol 3. ISH on paraffin-embedded tissue

Method

1. Stretch 4–6 μm paraffin sections on distilled water of 40 °C.

2. Pick up the sections on glutaraldehyde-activated poly-L-lysine-coated glass slides.

   Comments. If required, organosilane-coated slides can be used for better adhesion of the section. Reactive aldehyde groups remaining on the glass surface (after catching of sections on coated slides) can be blocked with 1% hydroxylammoniumchloride or 2% bovine serum albumin in PBS (1 h at 37 °C).

3. Air dry and bake the slides overnight at 56 °C.

4. Deparaffinize in 100% xylene (3 × 10 min).

5. Wash with 100% methanol (2 × 5 min).

6. Immerse slides in 1% H_2O_2 in 100% methanol (30 min).

7. Wash with 100% methanol (2 × 5 min).

8. Air dry.

9. If necessary the slides are immersed in 1 M NaSCN at 80 °C for 10 min to improve the efficiency of the proteolytic digestion step.

   Comments. Optimal tissue pre-treatment prior to ISH differs for each case. Thiocyanate has been shown to improve strongly the pepsin digestion. Optimization can be done on four sections, half of which are exposed to thiocyanate treatment. The non-thiocyanate sections are digested with pepsin for 15 and 30 min, while the thiocyanate-treated sections are digested for 5 and 15 min. On the basis of the ISH results on these sections a decision can be made about appropriate pre-treatment conditions. This may involve a shorter pepsin digestion time when (part of) the tissue morphology is lost. Conversely, when the tissue morphology seems to be unaffected by pepsin (after thiocyanate) a longer digestion time is used. Alternatively, protocols to improve efficiency of digestion involve: immersing slides in 0.2 M HCl for 20 min at room temperature or several cycles of freezing and thawing, microwaving, or putting in the pressure cooker (Wotherspoon, personal communication).

10. Wash with H_2O (2 × 5 min)

11. Incubate slides for 5–60 min at 37 °C in 4 mg pepsin(porcine stomach mucosa, 2500–3500 units per mg protein) per ml 0.2 M HCl.

    Comment. 30 min is standard. Pepsin in combination with HCl is recommended, although proteinase K (range 100–500 µg/ml 2 mM $CaCl_2$; 10 mM Tris HCl, pH 7.6, digestion time 10–30 min) and pronase could also be used for proteolytic digestion.

12. Rinse slides in H_2O (5 × dip washes) and PBS 5 × dip washes).

13. Slides are dehydrated in 70, 90, and 100% ethanol (3 min each).

14. Air dry.

    Comment. If required, for an adequate adhesion of the sections, slides can be baked for 30 min at 80 °C.

15. Apply the probe (1–3 ng/µl) in 10–15 µl hybridization buffer under a coverslip. Seal coverslip with rubber cement.

16. Denature slide at 80 °C for 4–10 min.

    Comment. 8 min at 80 °C is standard, denaturation at 90 °C in most cases results in loss of tissue material and/or nuclear morphology. A very mild denaturation procedure is based on the preparation of single-stranded DNA by enzymatic digestion of the double strand; in this case a heat denaturation can be avoided resulting in histological preservation (van Dekken *et al.* 1988; van Dekken *et al.* 1992a)

17. Hybridize in a moist chamber overnight at 37 °C.

Protocol 4. ISH on frozen tissue sections

Method

1. Stretch 4–6 µm frozen sections on poly-L-lysine (or organosilane)-coated glass slides.

2. Air dry overnight at room temperature.

3. Fix sections in methanol–acetone (1:1) for 20 min at −20 °C.

    Comment. Fixation of slides in 1% paraformaldehyde in PBS for 10 min at room temperature may be necessary if the morphology is lost during hybridization.

In situ *Hybridization*

4. Wash in PBS, 0.5% Tween (2 × 5 min).

5. Incubate slides for 10 min at 37°C in 50–400 μg pepsin (porcine stomach mucosa, 2500–3500 units per mg protein) per ml 0.01 M HCl. Optimum conditions should be determined.

   Comment. For a mild permeabilization slides can be immersed in 0.1 M HCl, 0.05 Triton X-100, or Tween-20 for 15 min.

6. Rinse slides in H_2O (5 × dip washes) and PBS (5 × dip washes).

7. Post-fix cells in 1% formaldehyde in PBS for 10 min at room temperature.

8. After fixation slides are rinsed in PBS (5 × dip washes) and H_2O (5 × dip washes).

9. Slides are dehydrated in 70, 90, and 100% ethanol (3 min each) and air-dried.

   Comment. If required for an adequate adhesion of cells, slides are baked for 30–60 min at 80°C.

10. Apply the probe (1–3 ng/μl) in hybridization buffer (5–10 μl) under a coverslip. Seal the coverslip with rubber cement (not mandatory).

11. Denature slides at 70–80°C for 2–4 min.

    Comment. 3 min at 70°C is standard. Probe and target DNA can be denatured separately. Target DNA is denatured by immersing the slides in 70% formamide, 2 × SSC for 3 min, slides are dehydrated in an ethanol series (4°C).

12. Hybridize in a moist chamber overnight at 37 °C.

8

Single and simultaneous nucleic acid detection in clinical samples

C.S. HERRINGTON

Introduction

In situ hybridization (ISH) may be defined as the direct detection of nucleic acids in cellular material. Its application to human pathology, therefore, involves the detection of both normal and abnormal nucleic acids in human cells and tissues (for review see Herrington and McGee, 1992a; Herrington 1994a). The development of techniques for ISH, in the context of pathology, has been directed towards procedures that are clinically useful. This requires not only the production of clinically relevant information, but also the ability to perform the procedures as part of a routine diagnostic service. A variety of cell and tissue samples can be studied using ISH, from individual chromosomes in metaphase spreads (Bhatt *et al.* 1988) to archival paraffin-embedded biopsy material (Chapter 7). Using appropriately labelled probes, the presence or absence of normal and abnormal nucleic acids can be detected and correlated with cell and tissue morphology. For many years, ISH was performed using isotopic probe labels for the detection of hybridized duplexes. However, these require autoradiographic detection techniques, which are time-consuming. More recently, isotopes of higher specific activity, which require shorter autoradiographic exposure times, have been used (e.g. ^{35}S) (see Chapter 5). A quicker and safer approach is to use non-isotopic probe labels, detected by histochemical means. This is termed nonisotopic *in situ* hybridization (NISH). Many different compounds have been used as probe labels (Herrington and McGee, 1992a; Hopman, 1995; Chapter 7) but the most widely used example is biotin (Langer *et al.* 1981). This was originally employed in NISH in order to utilize its high-affinity binding to the naturally occurring protein, avidin. Many different methods of detection have been developed, utilizing conjugates of avidin to both enzymes and fluorochromes. More recently, alternatives to biotin, the most popular of which is digoxigenin (Herrington *et al.* 1989a), have been explored in order to circumvent the problem of endogenous biotin, which is present in many tissues. In parallel, techniques have been developed for detection of more than one nucleic acid within individual cells. This has been achieved in isolated cells (Cremer *et al.* 1988; Hopman *et al.* 1988; Nederlof *et al.* 1989) using fluorescent detection systems that can be applied to the detection of up to 12 different colours simultaneously (Dauwerse *et al.* 1992). However, fluorescence-based procedures are less applicable to the analysis of archival material because of background autofluorescence, and hence non-fluorescent methods have been more commonly used in this context (Herrington *et al.* 1989a,b) (see below). This allows analysis of the relationship between nucleic acids within cells, in addition to the morphology of the tissue containing them. Similar considerations apply to simultaneous immunohistochemistry and *in situ* hybridization (see below).

NISH has been applied to the analysis of both human and non-human DNA in clinical biopsies (Herrington and McGee, 1992a; Hopman *et al.* 1992). The detection of human sequences in intact human cells has been termed interphase cytogenetics, which has been reviewed elsewhere (see Chapter 7; Herrington, 1994a). However, the flexibility and routine applicability of the techniques can be illustrated with reference to viral detection. The remainder of this chapter is therefore concerned with viral detection in clinical samples.

Viral detection in clinical samples

Introduction

The diagnosis of viral infection can often be inferred from clinical features. However, definite diagnosis requires either direct demonstration of the virus or its cytopathic effect, or detection of a specific immunological response. The latter, however, depends on the phase of infection, immunocompetence of the host, and assays for hormonal and/or cell-mediated immunity. In addition, widespread exposure of the population to certain types of virus, e.g. Epstein–Barr virus (EBV) can complicate diagnosis as only a specific IgM response is informative. Similarly, anamnestic rises in antibody titre can create diagnostic confusion. The direct demonstration of virus by viral culture or within tissues or body fluids provides a definite diagnosis. For some viruses, viral culture is either impossible (e.g. for human papillomaviruses; HPV) or technically time-consuming. Viruses can be demonstrated directly in human tissues in several ways. These include conventional histological staining, electron microscopy, and immunohistochemistry for viral antigens. The use of morphological criteria, that is the detection of the cytopathic effect of the virus, for the diagnosis of viral infection is non-specific and insensitive. For example, koilocytes are not indicative of infection by a particular type of (HPV) and, similarly, not all lesions containing HPCs show koilocytic atypia. Immunohistochemistry detects only the antigen to which the antibody is directed and does not detect virus that is not producing that antigen. CaSki cells, for example, which contain integrated HPV 16 sequences, do not express viral capsid protein and therefore do not stain with antibodies to that protein. Electron microscopy is useful for the diagnosis of specific lesions, e.g. atypical herpetic vesicular eruptions, but is only capable of detecting intact virions; additionally, viral subtypes, e.g. of HPV or herpesviruses, look the same and are therefore indistinguishable.

Viruses are generally defined, classified, and typed according to their nucleic acid content. The detection of nucleic acid in clinical material is therefore the most appropriate way of achieving a clinical diagnosis and of investigating the epidemiology and natural history of viral infections. Nucleic acids can be analysed in two ways: after extraction from tissue with or without amplification by the polymerase chain reaction (see below), or directly by *in situ* hybridization. In the remainder of this chapter, only *in situ* hybridization and the recently described combination of ISH and PCR will be discussed.

Viruses may contain DNA or RNA, but never both. DNA may be double- or single-stranded and RNA sense or antisence. Finally, an RNA virus may replicate via a double-stranded DNA intermediate. Many viruses have now been investigated using ISH (Syrjänen, 1992). Those receiving the most attention have been the DNA viruses: HPV (Syrjanen *et al.* 1988; Herrington *et al.* 1995a), herpesviruses [EBV, HSV (human sarcoma virus), CMV cytomegalovirus)] (Burns *et al.* 1986; Wolber and Lloyd 1988), and polyomaviruses (JC, BK) (Boerman *et al.* 1989), which are double-stranded; parvoviruses (Porter *et al.* 1988), which are single-stranded; and hepatitis B virus (Blum *et al.* 1983), which has a mixed double- and single-stranded genome. Most DNA viruses replicate within the cell nucleus (the notable exception being pox viruses) and the nucleic acid may remain separate from the host genome, i.e. episomal, or may integrate into one or more chromosomes. The difference can be detected by *in situ* hybridization through differences in signal morphology (see below). Episomal viruses are replicating and are therefore present in large numbers. This facilitates their detection by *in situ* hybridization. However, integrated viruses may be present in very low numbers and therefore require sensitive procedures for their detection. The sensitivity of the non-fluorescent, non-isotopic procedure we use routinely is approximately 2.5–12 copies of HPV, which is equivalent to approximately 20–100 kb of target sequence (Herrington *et al.* 1991). Using the same technique, a single copy of the EBV genome was detected in paraffin-embedded material using a probe for the *Bam*H1 repeat, which is approximately 40 kb in length (Coates *et al.* 1991). By amplifying this detection system, single copy HPV infection was detectable in cell lines (Herrington *et al.* 1992a) but this method was not found to be routinely applicable to either cytological or histological material because of high background staining. Another approach to the problem of low copy number is the detection of virus-specific mRNA, which is not only specific for the virus but also for the phase of infection. This is particularly useful for the detection of Epstein–Barr virus, the demonstration of EBER RNA being routinely applicable (Zhou *et al.* 1994).

RNA viruses are also detectable by NISH (Haase *et al.* 1985a; Haase 1986), but these have received less attention than DNA viruses. The intact virion of oncornaviruses contains single-stranded RNA, but a double-stranded DNA intermediate is formed during replication. The intermediate integrates into the host genome and has been implicated in oncogenesis. HIV-1 (human immunodeficiency virus) belongs to this group of viruses and has been investigated by NISH (Pezzella *et al.* 1987).

A more recent modification of the *in situ* hybridization technique is its combination with polymerase chain reaction amplification of the target DNA. There are two basic approaches to this combination of PCR and *in situ* hybridization: amplification of the target sequence with direct incorporation of label molecules into the product (*in situ* PCR); and prior amplification of target DNA followed by conventional *in situ* hybridization using a labelled probe (PCR *in situ* hybridization). There are reports of success with this technique, many of which involve the demonstration of HPV and HIV sequences (Haase *et al.* 1990; Nuovo *et al.* 1991; O'Leary *et al.* 1995, 1996). Technically, these procedures are capricious and reproducibility is a problem. However, several studies have been reported in which the target sequences have been retained within the nucleus after amplification allowing subsequent detection by *in situ* hybridization (Nuovo *et al.* 1991; Komminoth *et al.* 1992).

HPVs have been extensively investigated by all the methods described above and illustrate the ways in which NISH can be used in this context. Therefore, the detection of HPV in biopsies and cytopathological smears will be used as illustrative examples. Practical details of the combination of PCR and *in situ* hybridization are given in Nuovo *et al.* (1991) and O'Leary *et al.* (1995).

HPV detection in archival material

Papillomaviruses have been detected in most lesions of squamous epithelia (Syrjanen 1987). They are known to integrate into the host genome (Cooper *et al.* 1991a; Cullen *et al.* 1991) and have been implicated in the aetiology of many squamous cell carcinomata, particularly that of the uterine cervix (Herrington 1994b; Herrington *et al.* 1995a,b). The virus is easily detectable by *in situ* hybridization in benign, premalignant, and malignant lesions of many sites and it has been noted that the morphological characteristics of episomal virus disappear with progression of morphology from benign to malignant. This has been taken to imply integration of the viral genome, an interpretation that is supported by the association of viral integration with high grade CIN and invasive squamous cell carcinoma (Cooper *et al.* 1991a,b,c).

In situ hybridization allows correlation of the presence of virus with the morphology of infected tissues. By using specific probes, viral subtypes can be distinguished and the precise infecting species found. This has considerable epidemiological importance as well as relevance for the natural history of HPV infections. Thus, it has been shown that HPV1 is associated with benign cutaneous lesions, and several other less common HPV types with the rare premalignant syndrome epidermodysplasia verruciformis (Pfister and Fuchs 1987). Similarly, HPV 6 and 11 are found in benign anogenital lesions and HPV 16, 18, 31, 33, and 35 in premalignant and malignant lesions of both male and female genitalia (Pfister and Fuchs 1987). The strength of these associations has led to the definition of 'high' (HPV 16 and 18 particularly), 'intermediate' (HPV 31, 33, and 35 particularly), and 'low' (HPV 6 and 11 particularly) risk types (Lorincz *et al.* 1992).

The investigation of archival biopsies requires accessibility of target nucleic acid for hybridization with molecular probes. This requires initial dewaxing of sections by conventional means, followed by proteolysis to remove both viral and cellular proteins, which impede diffusion of the probe and access of the probe to the target. This process is termed unmasking and has been performed with a variety of enzymes. These enzymes vary in potency, not only from type to type but also from manufacturer to manufacturer. Thus, conditions must be optimized using enzymes from one supplier. Initially, pepsin–HCl was thought to be the most appropriate enzyme for unmasking HPV (Burns *et al.* 1987), primarily as the use of more potent enzymes led to an unacceptable rate of detachment of sections from slides. The use of aminopropyltriethoxysilane as a section adhesive (Burns *et al.* 1988) has allowed the use of higher concentrations of proteinase K (up to 1mg/ml), producing significantly more effective unmasking. This is now the method used by several groups for HPV sequences (Wells *et al.* 1987; Burns *et al.* 1988; Syrjanen 1992). However, this does not imply general utility for nucleic acid unmasking: the detection of chromosome-specific repeat probes is optimum with pepsin–HCl (Hopman *et al.* 1992; Chapter 7). Thus, unmasking procedures must be optimized for each experimental system.

Having exposed the sequence of interest, appropriately labelled probe(s) (see Chapter 3) is added and the tissue section and probe simultaneously denatured by heat. The addition of exogenous unlabelled human or salmon sperm DNA in excess is often necessary to reduce non-specific staining, but has not been found beneficial for the detection of HPV in archival biopsies (see Appendix). Hybridization is then allowed to occur under appropriate conditions (for a full discussion see Herrington and McGee 1992a). Following hybridization, excess probe is removed and mismatched hybrids dissociated using appropriate salt, formamide, and temperature combinations to a predetermined level of stringency (see Chapter 1 and Herrington *et al.* 1990, 1993, 1995a). After a blocking step, probe–target hybrids are detected by non-fluorescent histochemical means.

The detection systems employed depend on the reporter molecule to be detected. Most reporters (e.g. digoxigenin, acetylaminofluorene, mercury) are detected using specific antibodies, but biotin can be visualized using either antibody- or avidin-based systems. Single step detection requires the linkage of antibody or avidin to an indicator enzyme: the most widely used examples are horseradish peroxidase and alkaline phosphatase. Amplified detection systems employ a variety of mechanisms to enhance the signal and hence sensitivity and will be discussed below. Several substrates of different colours can be used for each of these enzymes and can be manipulated to allow either appropriate counterstaining or a combination for multiple labelling (see below).

The sensitivity of a particular non-fluorescent detection system depends on several parameters: the availability of target sequences for hybridization, i.e. unmasking; the type of probe; the reporter molecule used; the affinity of the antibody/avidin for the reporter; the degree of amplification by multiple antibody/avidin/enzyme layers; and the enzyme/chromogen combination. The investigation of the contribution of each of these factors to sensitivity requires that all other parameters are comparable.

The probes used for NISH are generally of three main types: nick translated, random-primed, and oligonucleotide. Nick translated probes are the most widely used as they are simple to produce and use. As the labelling method (see Chapter 3) introduces nicks at random into the double-stranded DNA molecule, labelled fragments of different length and containing variable proportions of insert and vector are produced. It has been suggested that these fragments anneal together via their overlapping portions to produce a probe network, thereby amplifying the target sequence '*in situ*'. The same arguments apply to probes generated by random-primed synthesis, but not to oligonucleotide probes. In addition, individual oligonucleotides, being shorter than other probes, are likely to be less sensitive than their nick translated and random-primed counterparts. However, oligonucleotides are naturally more specific and can be used individually or in combination. The type of probe should therefore be chosen to suit the experimental system under study.

The affinity of the detector molecule for the reporter also contributes to sensitivity: the high affinity of avidin for biotin was one reason why this molecule was chosen as a non-isotopic probe label (Langer *et al.* 1981). The maximum affinity of antibodies for antigen ($K_d = 10^{-12}$) is approximately 1000 times less than that of avidin for biotin ($K_d = 10^{-15}$). The sensitivity of single step detection of digoxigenin-labelled probes was found to be less than that of a corresponding system for the detection of biotin (Herrington *et al.* 1989a). However, digoxigenin was detected using an antibody conjugate, whereas biotin was detected using the avidin conjugate, as shown in Fig. 8.1a. The use of three-step amplification systems (Fig. 8.1b) employing monoclonal antibodies for both digoxigenin and biotin and the same second and third steps (see Appendix), renders digoxigenin more sensitive, largely because of lower background staining and better spatial resolution of the signal (Herrington *et al.* 1991).

Amplification of detection can be achieved by either antibody layering techniques (Fig. 8.1b) or by enzyme/antibody complexes (Fig. 8.1c), which increase the number of enzyme molecules bound to each reporter molecule.

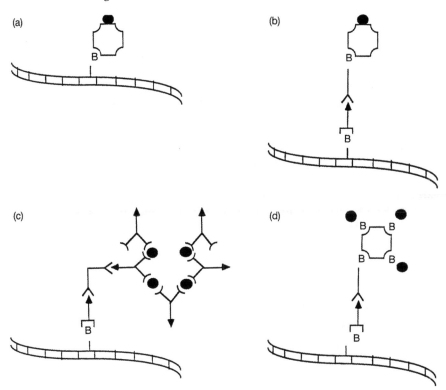

Fig. 8.1. (a) Single-step detection of biotin (B). Biotin is detected using a conjugate of alkaline phosphatase (●) and avidin(◯). (b) Three-step detection of digoxigenin (D). A monoclonal antibody into digoxigenin (⊐➤) is linked via biotinylated rabbit anti-mouse immunoglobulin (B—≺) to an avidin–alkaline phosphatase conjugate. This combines the high specificity of the monoclonal antibody with the high sensitivity interaction between avidin and biotin. (c) Alkaline phosphatase anti-alkaline phosphatase (APAAP) detection. A monoclonal antibody to digoxigenin (D) is detected using rabbit anti-mouse immuno-globulin. The second valency of this molecule is then used to bind to the pre-formed APAAP complex. The APAAP complex is produced by mixing alkaline phosphatase (●) with monoclonal anti-alkaline phosphatase (⟩➤). (d) Avidin-biotinylated alkaline phosphatase complex (ABC). In this method, digoxigenin is detected using a combination of antibody and enzyme amplification. Antibody to biotin is detected using a biotinylated second antibody followed by a pre-formed complex of avidin with biotinylated alkaline phosphatase (B●). This combines the high affinity of the avidin–biotin interaction with occupancy of the four binding sites of avidin for biotin.

Thus, the combination of monoclonal antibody to the reporter molecule (e.g. monoclonal anti-digoxin used in the Appendix) linked via a biotinylated linker antibody to an avidin conjugate produces high specificity (monoclonal antibody) and sensitivity (avidin conjugate). Alternatively, monoclonal anti-bodies to reporter molecules can be linked through rabbit anti-mouse immunoglobulin to a complex of detector enzyme and antibody to the detector enzyme [e.g. peroxidase anti-peroxidase (PAP) and alkaline phosphatase anti-alkaline phosphatase (APAAP)] (Sternberger *et al.* 1970; Cordell *et al.* 1984). The two approaches of antibody and enzyme enhancement are combined in methods based on the avidin biotinylated alkaline phosphatase complex (ABC) initially proposed for avidin biotinylated peroxidase by HSU *et al.* (1981) for the detection of antigen. These methods also exploit the tetravalency of avidin. Methods b–d, shown in Fig. 8.1, can be modified for the detection of other reporter molecules by using the appropriate primary antibody and can be manipulated to produce combined detection systems of great flexibility. Sensitivity depends also on the choice of chromogenic enzymes and substrates: alkaline phosphatase-based systems tend to be of greater sensitivity than those employing peroxidase unless enhanced substrates, e.g. metal-chelated DAB (Hsu and Soban 1982; Heryet and Gatter 1992) are used. Similarly, silver enhancement of diaminobenzidine (DAB) significantly increases the sensitivity of peroxidase-based detection of sequences in archival material (Burns *et al.* 1987).

Measurement of the sensitivity of detection systems is not easy. Relative sensitivity can be assessed by estimation of the number of positive cells within a given area of comparable tissue sections using different systems. Absolute sensitivity can only be estimated by analysing the ability of particular systems to detect sequences of known copy number. This has been performed using cell lines containing multiple copies of HPVs, for example CaSki, HeLa, and SiHa cells. Syrjanen *et al.* (1988) estimated the sensitivity of biotinylated probes to be 10–50 copies based on their ability to detect HPV consistently in CaSki and HeLa, but not SiHa, cells. However, the copy number is likely to vary from cell to cell and therefore a more appropriate method of estimation is to analyse the frequency distribution of signals within these cells (for example, see Fig. 8.2) and compare the median of the distribution with the average copy number per cell derived by dot blot hybridization (Herrington *et al.* 1989a). This approach gave a sensitivity of approximately 30 copies per cell for single step detection methods, and 2.5–12 copies per cell for amplified detection systems (Herrington *et al.* 1991). Further amplification of detection allowed the detection of single copy HPV in SiHa cells using digoxigenin-labelled probes, but this was not found to be applicable to routine material (Herrington *et al.* 1992a).

The three-step detection method described here for digoxigenin-labelled probes is useful for the rapid screening of tissue blocks for the presence of HPV infection as it allows correlation of the signal with tissue morphology. This method has been found to be particularly useful in the analysis of signal morphology within individual cells since the higher resolution of peroxidase-based detection systems allows easier distinction between punctate and diffuse signals (Cooper *et al.* 1991a,b,c). Although this approach is intrinsically less sensitive than using alkaline phosphatase-based systems, in our hands the

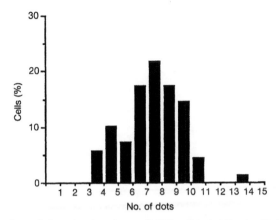

Fig. 8.2. The number of discrete signals per CaSki cell hybridized with biotinylated HPV 14 probe has been plotted against the percentage of cells. The distribution of dot number in 80 cells is skewed, with a median of eight dots per cell. The copy number of mid log phase CaSki cells was estimated to be 270 by dot blot hybridization. This gives a sensitivity of approximately 30 copies.

latter give less interpretable results (Herrington *et al.* 1991, 1992a). The distinction of punctate and diffuse signals has been shown to discriminate between episomal and integrated HPV sequences (Cooper *et al.* 1991a,b,c) in cervical intraepithelial neoplasia and in invasive cervical carcinoma: this approach provides a simple method for the determination of the physical state of viral sequences without a requirement for nucleic acid extraction techniques.

NISH analysis allows the individual identification of HPV subtypes in clinical biopsies and hence the distinction of 'low', 'intermediate', and 'high' risk viral subtypes. The application of these methods to archival biopsy files has provided a wealth of retrospective information regarding HPV infection of human tissues (Fig. 8.3; Herrington 1994b; Herrington *et al.* 1995c).

Analysis of cervical smears

Although the analysis of cervical biopsies by NISH is useful in the investigation of HPV infection, the necessary prerequisite for this analysis is that the patient has had a cervical biopsy. However, cervical screening for premalignant lesions involves the collection of cervical smears, which are analysed cytologically for the presence of abnormal cells indicative of cervical intraepithelial neoplasia. The detection of HPV DNA in cervical smears has posed several problems. First, only one smear is usually taken and this is naturally required for cytopathological diagnosis. It is thus impossible to perform controls on material from the same patient. With the introduction of methods for preparing monolayers from a single sample, this problem may be

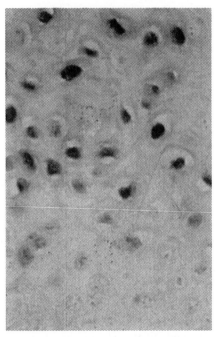

Fig. 8.3. A section from a formalin-fixed, paraffin-embedded condyloma acuminatum was hybridized with an HPV 6 probe. Clear nuclear signal can be seen (see plate section).

solved as more monolayers are clinically used. Secondly, cervical smears contain a variable amount of mucin and are contaminated with bacteria, fungi, and protozoa. This may lead to technical problems, particularly high background staining.

HPV infection of exfoliated cells has been analysed by a variety of methods. The analysis of smears from normal women by Southern blotting suggested that 11–12% of normal smears harboured HPV sequences (Lorincz *et al.* 1986; Toon *et al.* 1986). 'Filter *in situ* hybridization' has provided evidence in agreement with this (Wagner *et al.* 1984) but a large study of 1930 normal smears showed that only 1% of these samples contained HPV sequences (Melchers *et al.* 1989), with 100% concordance between filter *in situ* hybridization and Southern blot analysis. A study by *in situ* hybridization, in which the sensitivity was estimated to be 50–100 copies, found that 15.4% of normal smears contained HPV sequences and the percentage positivity increased with increasing abnormality to a maximum of 78.2% for CIN 3 (Pao *et al.* 1989). Use of the more sensitive system (approximately 2.5–12 copies per cell) described in the Appendix (Fig. 8.4, and see Herrington and McGee 1992b) found HPV sequences in 30–35% of smears taken from patients with normal cervical cytology, including a group of patients from a sexually transmitted disease clinic (Herrington *et al.* 1992a; Troncone *et al.* 1992) and

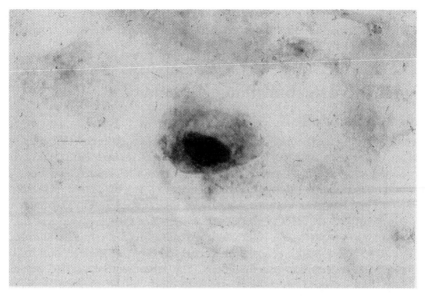

Fig. 8.4. Hybridization of a cervical smear with a cocktail of biotinylated probes for HPV 6, 11, 16, 18, 31, 33, 35. Clear nuclear signal can be seen in both nuclei of a binucleate koilocyte (see plate section).

direct comparison of this NISH system with 'Virapap', which is a modification of filter *in situ* hybridization, showed that NISH was of significantly greater diagnostic sensitivity (Troncone *et al.* 1992).

Polymerase chain reaction amplification of HPV DNA has been employed extensively since 1989 and formal comparison with NISH has shown that PCR has greater diagnostic sensitivity (Herrington *et al.* 1995a). Moreover, despite early studies that suggested that a high proportion of apparently normal cervical smears contained HPV sequences as determined by PCR, more recent data has shown that a high rate of false positive results is obtained with this technique if measures are not taken to eliminate or control for sample contamination (Shibata 1992). Recent PCR-based estimates of the prevalence of HPV in such patients range from 3.5–30% (Schiffman, 1992' Walboomers *et al.* 1992) and demonstrate that the prevalence of HPV is age dependent (Melkert 1993; Herrington *et al.* 1996). The figures obtained depend in part on the population studied, but there does appear to be a difference between patients with normal and dyskaryotic smears, and a recent PCR-based case–control study suggests that the majority of all grades of CIN can be attributed to HPV infection (Schiffman *et al.* 1993).

However, the use of semi-quantitative PCR techniques has shown a relationship between higher amounts of 'intermediate' and 'high' risk HPV DNA and CIN 2 or 3 (Cuzick *et al.* 1992, 1994; Bavin *et al.* 1993) and it has been suggested, therefore, that less sensitive techniques may be more applicable in determining patients with more significant cervical disease. Studies utilizing *in situ* hybridization have confirmed this association (Herrington *et al.* 1992b, 1995b).

Combined detection of nucleic acids

Introduction

Techniques for the histochemical detection of two antigens (Wagner *et al.* 1988), or antigen and nucleic acid (Wolber and Lloyd 1988), have been described and the simultaneous detection of two nucleic acids has been performed by isotopic *in situ* hybridization using two isotopic labels (Haase *et al.* 1985b). This, however, requires the use of differential autoradiography with its attendant lack of cellular resolution. It also has the disadvantage that the operator waits weeks for a result and is exposed to a dual radiation hazard. The use of non-isotopic reporter molecules allows probe detection by both fluorescent and non-fluorescent means. The latter can be carried out more quickly than isotopic procedures, are safe, and can be manipulated in the context of dual labelling to produce fluorescence signals and substrate products of contrasting colours.

The simultaneous detection of two nucleic acids can be accomplished in two ways: sequential hybridization and detection of probes labelled with the same reporter molecule; or simultaneous hybridization and detection of probes labelled with different reporters. The former approach is more time-consuming and employs many more practical steps, leading to higher background noise. Although useful in some circumstances (Herrington 1994a), the use of more than one reporter molecule is more appropriate.

The gold standard by which alternative DNA reporters are judged is biotin. This was originally employed in NISH in order to utilize its binding with high affinity to the naturally occurring protein avidin (Langer *et al.* 1981). Many alternatives have been developed and those most frequently used to date have been aceylaminofluorene (AAF) and mercury (Hopman *et al.* 1988). These have been detected primarily by fluorescent methods and have been used to visualize chromosome-specific sequences in isolated cells (Cremer *et al.* 1988; Hopman *et al.* 1988; Nederlof *et al.* 1989; Chapter 7). More recently, two approaches have been described for the combination of reporter molecules within individual probes. The first is combinatorial labelling, where probes are labelled with two or more fluorochromes in approximately equimolar ratios, e.g. three fluorochromes give seven possible different probes (label 1 alone, label 2 alone, label 3 alone, labels 1 and 2, labels 1 and 3, labels 2 and 3, and labels 1, 2, and 3 together) and analysis is carried out using a cooled, charged, coupled device (CCD) camera and image analysis (Ried *et al.* 1992). The alternative is known as ratio labelling, where probes labelled with different reporter molecules are mixed in different ratios to give different colours:

three labels have been used to paint chromosomes in 12 different colours, which are real and so do not require image analysis (Dauwerse *et al.* 1992). However, NISH on paraffin sections is best performed using non-fluorescent detection of probe labels since fluorescent methods are less suitable because of tissue autofluorescence. Multiple probe detection is therefore limited by the ability to produce chromogens of sufficiently different optical character-istics to allow distinction by transmitted light: this generally restricts the number of probes detectable to two (Hopman *et al.* 1988; Herrington *et al.* 1989b).

The most commonly used alternative to biotin is digoxigenin, which is the aglycone derivative of digoxin. Antibodies to digoxin have been shown to cross-react with it with high affinity (Smith *et al.* 1970; Monji *et al.* 1980; Valdes *et al.* 1984) and therefore the well-established antisera used in the assessment and treatment of digoxin toxicity can be applied to the detection of digoxigenin in NISH. Probes labelled with digoxigenin have been shown to be as sensitive as biotin when detected by compatible non-fluorescent means (Herrington *et al.* 1989a) and these two reporters therefore provide suitable alternatives in NISH.

Dual *in situ* hybridization

The method described in the Appendix allows the simultaneous non-fluor-escent detection of two nucleic acids in contrasting colours in clinical biopsies and cervical smears. It is easy, quick, and reliable. The whole procedure, from section cutting or smear fixation to probe visualization, can be completed in approximately 5 h. This is only 30 mins longer than the detection of one nucleic acid. By mixing probes labelled with digoxigenin and biotin, this technique allows denaturation and hybridization to be performed simultane-ously with the target DNA. The detection of biotin using a streptavidin conjugate, and of digoxigenin using an alkaline phosphatase conjugate, allows mixing of the two detection systems, without cross-reaction, and simultaneous application to the tissue section. The peroxidase substrate (AEC), used to detect biotin-labelled probes, produces a red product and therefore the digoxigenin-labelled probe was detected using a blue substrate (NBT/BCIP) for alkaline phosphatase. Incubation in substrates is performed sequentially, since peroxidase and alkaline phosphatase have different pH optima.

This system for biopsies was developed for the simultaneous detection of the Y chromosome and HPV (Fig. 8.5) (Herrington *et al.* 1989b) and has been applied without modification to the simultaneous detection of two subtypes of HPV (Fig. 8.6) (Herrington *et al.* 1990; Herrington, 1997). It is probable that its application to other nucleic acid sequences, which produce NISH signals of different morphology, will require the probe labelling strategy and substrate incubation times to be determined by experiment. It is important that the two systems used for double labelling are of equivalent sensitivity, particularly if

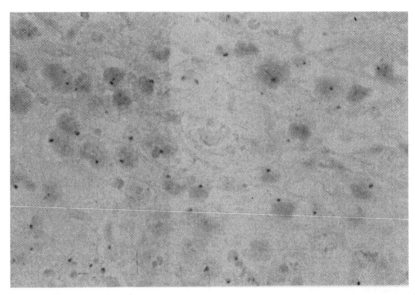

Fig. 8.5. Dual nucleic acid detection: biotinylated HPV 6 probe and digoxigenin-labelled Y chromosome-specific probe were hybridized to a section from a male condyloma acuminatum. The HPV signal can be seen as red and the Y signal as blue dots (see plate section).

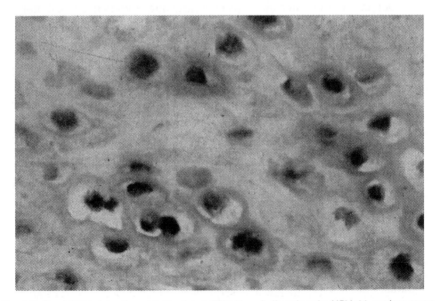

Fig. 8.6. Dual HPV detection: biotinylated HPV 6 and digoxigenin HPV 11 probes were hybridized to a section from a condyloma acuminatum under conditions of low stringency and detected to produce colours as for Fig 8.5. The signal from both probes can be seen within the same nucleus (see plate section).

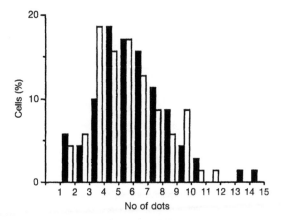

Fig. 8.7. The frequency distribution of the number of dots per cell for the two detection systems used for dual nucleic acid detection are shown. Open columns represent the detection of biotinylated probes with streptavidin peroxidase–AEC and shaded columns the detection of digoxigenin-labelled probes using NBT/BCIP.

the signals being detected are of similar morphology, in order that the signals generated are directly comparable in all respects other than colour. This has been shown to be the case for the system described here by analysing the frequency distribution (see Fig. 8.7) of the number of dots produced by both systems in CaSki cells (Herrington *et al*. 1989a). Where the target sequences are present in significantly different numbers or are of different length, detection of biotin-labelled probes can be amplified to enhance the signal by comparison with that generated by the digoxigenin-labelled probe: this has been used in the analysis of dual HPV infection (Herrington 1992).

Application to cervical smears

As has been mentioned previously, the analysis of cervical smears by NISH is complicated by the lack of duplicated specimens from each patient. In general, this has led to the use of cocktails of probes, containing probes for each of the HPV subtypes found in anogenital lesions. Alternatively, cervicovaginal lavage can be used to produce cellular suspensions that can be used to produce multiple smears (Pao *et al*. 1989). However, each smear produced by this method is unlikely to represent an adequate sample of the whole cervix and, more importantly, the collection of such samples is expensive in terms of both time and equipment. By labelling HPV 6 and 11 with biotin and HPV 16, 18, 31, 33, and 35 with digoxigenin, the double detection system described for archival biopsies can be applied to cervical smears. This method was applied to a series of cervical smears, with red signal indicative of 'low' risk and blue signal of 'high' risk HPV infection (Fig. 8.8). By this means, 'low' risk HPV types were found in 21% and 'intermediate' and 'high' risk types in 25% of 128 smears taken from patients with normal cervical cytology taken

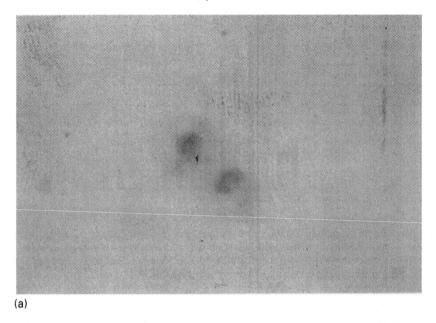

(a)

(b)

Fig. 8.8. The application of the dual detection system to cervical smears produces a red signal (a) indicative of HPV 6/11 infection and a blue signal (b) indicative of HPV 16/18/31/33/35 infection (see text and plate section).

from a sexually transmitted disease clinic (Herrington *et al.* 1992c). In the same study, 'low' risk HPV types were found in 26% and 'intermediate' and 'high' risk in 58% of 50 smears showing morphological changes of HPV infection.

Conclusion

In conclusion, *in situ* hybridization can be used to analyse the presence or absence of nucleic acids in a variety of cell and tissue samples. *In situ* hybridization is the only means by which a definite diagnosis of viral infection can be made in conjunction with the analysis of the morphology of the infected tissue. The methods described here are easy and quick and can be applied to the rapid screening of archival and current tissue blocks, thus providing a wealth of epidemiological data about oncogenic infectious disease. Although the sensitivity of methods currently available is limited, it is likely that low copy number sequences will soon be detectable in archival biopsies. The simultaneous detection of two nucleic acids on the same section and in the same nucleus in archival samples has allowed the investigation of double viral infection. Its application to other areas, for example the field of interphase cytogenetics, will allow the investigation of the relationship between nucleic acids in individual nuclei in archival material. Similarly, the application of these systems to the analysis of cervical smears will allow more effective HPV typing together with correlation with morphology.

References

Bancroft, J.D., and Stevens, A. (eds) (1977). *Theory and practice of histological techniques*. Churchill Livingstone, Edinburgh.

Bavin, P.J., Giles, J.A., Deery, A. *et al.* (1993). Use of semi-quantitative PCR for human papillomavirus DNA type 16 to identify women with high grade cervical disease in a population presenting with a mildly dyskaryotic smear report. *Br. J. Cancer*, **67**, 602–5.

Bhatt, B., Burns, J., Flannery, D., and McGee, J.O'D. (1988). Direct visualisation of single copy genes on banded metaphase chromosomes by nonisotopic *in situ* hybridisation. *Nucl. Acids Res.*, **16**, 3951–61.

Blum, H.E., Stowring, L., Figus, A., Montgomery, C.K., Haase, A.T., and Vyas, G.N. (1983). Detection of hepatitis B virus DNA in hepatocytes, bile duct epithelium and vascular elements by *in situ* hybridisation. *Proc. Natl. Acad. Sci. USA*, **80**, 6685–8.

Boerman, R.H., Arnoldous, E.P.J., Raap, A.K., Peters, A.C.B., Ter Schegget, J., and Van Der Ploeg, M. (1989). Diagnosis of progressive multifocal leucoencephalopathy by hybridisation techniques. *J. Clin. Pathol.*, **42**, 153–61.

Burns, J., Redfern, D.R.M., Esiri, M.M., and McGee, J.O'D. (1986). Human and viral gene detection in routine paraffin embedded tissue by *in situ* hybridisation with biotinylated probes: viral localisation in herpes encephalitis. *J. Clin. Pathol.*, **39**, 1066–73.

Burns, J., Graham, A.K., Frank, C., Fleming, K.A., Evans, M.F., and McGee, J.O'D. (1987). Detection of low copy human papilloma virus DNA and mRNA in routine paraffin sectins of cervix by non-isotopic *in situ* hybridisation. *J. Clin. Pathol.*, **40**, 858–64.

Burns, J., Graham, A.K., and McGee, J.O'D. (1988). Non-isotopic detection of *in situ* nucleic acid in cervix: an updated protocol. *J. Clin. Pathol.*, **41**, 897–9.

Coates, P.J., Mak, W.P., Slavin, G., and d'Ardenne, J. (1991). Detection of single copies of Epstein–Barr virus in paraffin wax sections by non-radioactive *in situ* hybridisation. *J. Clin. Pathol.*, **44**, 487–91.

Cooper, K., Herrington, C.S., Stickland, J.E., Evans, M.F., and McGee, J.O'D. (1991a). Episomal and integrated HPV in cervical neoplasia demonstrated by nonisotopic *in situ* hybridisation. *J. Clin. Pathol.*, **44**, 990–6.

Cooper, K., Herrington, C.S., Graham, A.K., Evans, M.F., and McGee, J.O'D. (1991b). *In situ* human papillomavirus (HPV) genotyping of cervical intraepithalial neoplasia in South African and British patients: evidence for putative HPV integration *in vivo. J. Clin. Pathol.*, **44**, 400–5.

Cooper, K., Herrington, C.S., Graham, A.K., Evans, M.F., and McGee, J.O'D. (1991c) *In situ* evidence for HPV 16, 18, 33 integration in cervical squamous cell cancer in Britain and South Africa. *J. Clin. Pathol.*, **44**, 406–9.

Cordell, J.L., Falini, B., Erber, W.N., Ghosh, A.K., Abdulaziz, Z., MacDonald, S., Pulford, K.A.F., Stein, H., and Mason, D.Y. (1984). Immunoenzymatic labelling of monoclonal antibodies using immune complexes of alkaline phosphatase and monoclonal anti-alkaline phosphatase (APAAP complexes). *J. Histochem. Cytochem.*, **32**, 219–29.

Cremer, T., Tesin, D., Hopman, A.H.N., and Manuelidis, L. (1988). Rapid interphase and metaphase assessment of specific chromosomal changes in neuroectodermal cells by *in situ* hybridisation with chemically modified DNA probes. *Exp. Cell. Res.*, **176**, 199–220.

Cullen, A.P., Reid, R., Campion, M., and Lorincz, A.T. (1991). Analysis of the physical state of different human papillomavirus DNAs in intraepithelial and invasive cervical neoplasia. *J. Virol.*, **65**, 606–12.

Cuzick, J., Terry, G., Ho, L., Hollingworth, T., and Anderson, M. (1992). Human papillomavirus type 16 in cervical smears as predictor of high-grade cervical intraepithelial neoplasia. *Lancet*, **339**, 959–60.

Cuzick, J., Terry, G., Ho, L., Hollingworth, T., and Anderson, M. (1994). Type-specific human papillomavirus DNA in abnormal smears as a predictor of high-grade cervical intraepithelial neoplasia. *Br. J. Cancer.*, **69**, 167–71.

Dauwerse, J.G., Wiegant, J., Raap, A.K., Breuning, M.H., and van Ommen, G. (1992). Multiople colors by fluorescence *in situ* hybridization using radio-labelled DNA probes create a molecular karyotype. *Hum. Mol. Genet.*, **1**, 593–8.

Haase, A.T. (1986). Analysis of viral infections by *in situ* hybridisation. *J. Histochem. Cytochem.*, **34**, 27–32.

Haase, A.T., Gantz, D., Eble, B. *et al.* (1985a). Natural history of restricted synthesis and expression of measles virus genes in subacute sclerosing panencephalitis. *Proc. Natl. Acad. Sci. USA*, **82**, 3020–4.

Haase, A.T., Walker, D., Ventura, P. *et al.* (1985b). Detection of two viral genomes in single cells by double-label hybridisation *in situ* and color microradioautography. *Science*, **227**, 189–92.

Haase, A.T., Retzel, E.F., and Staskus, K.A. (1990). Amplification and detection of lentiviral DNA inside cells. *Proc. Natl. Acad. Sci. USA*, **87**, 4971–5.

Herrington, C.S. (1992). Differentiation of viral and chromosomal nucleic acids in nuclei. In: *Non-radioactive labelling and detection of biomolecules*, (ed. C. Kessler), Springer-Verlag.

Herrington, C.S. (1994a). Interphase cytogenetics: principles and practice. *J. Histotechnol.*, **17**, 219–34.

Herrington, C.S. (1994b). Human papillomaviruses and cervical neoplasia I: classification, virology, pathology and epidemiology. *J. Clin. Pathol.*, **47**, 1066–72.

Herrington, C.S. (1997). Differentiation of viral and chromosomal nucleic acids in nuclei. In: *Non-radioactive labelling and detection of biomolecules*, (2nd edn), (ed. C. Kessler). Springer-Verlag, Berlin.

Herrington, C.S. and McGee, J.O'D. (1992a). Principles and basic methodology of DNA/RNA detection by *in situ* hybridisation. In: *Diagnostic molecule pathology. A practical approach*, Vol. 1, pp. 69–102. Oxford University Press, Oxford.

Herrington, C.S. and McGee, J.O'D. (ed.) (1992b). *In situ* hybridisation in diagnostic cytopathology. In: *Diagnostic molecular pathology. A practical approach*, Vol. 1, pp. 205–20. Oxford University Press, Oxford.

Herrington, C.S. and McGee, J'O'D. (1994). Discrimination of closely homologous human genomic and viral sequences in cells and tissues: further characteristisation of Tm^l. *Histochem. J.*, **26**, 545–52.

Herrington, C.S., Burns, J., Graham, A.K., Evans, M.F., and McGee, J.O'D. (1989a). Interphase cytogenetics using biotin and digoxigenin labelled probes I: relative sensitivity of both reporters for detection of HPV16 in CaSki cells. *J. Clin. Pathl.*, **42**, 592–600.

Herrington, C.S., Burns, J., Graham, A.K., Bhatt, B., and McGee, J.O'D. (1989b). Interphase cytogenetics using biotin and digoxigenin labelled probes II: simultaneous detection of two nucleic acid species in individual nuclei. *J. Clin. Pathol.*, **42**, 601–6.

Herrington, C.S., Burns, J., Graham, A.J., and McGee, J.O'D. (1990). Discrimination of closely homologous HPV types by nonisotopic *in situ* hybridization: definition and derivation of tissue melting temperatures. *Histochem. J.*, **22**, 545–54.

Herrington, C.S., Graham, A.K., and McGee, J. O'D. (1991). Interphase cytogenetics using biotin and digoxigenin labelled probes III: increased sensitivity and flexibility for detecting HPV in cervical biopsy specimens and cell lines. *J. Clin. Pathol.*, **44**, 33–8.

Herrington, C.S., de Angelis, M., Evans, M.F., Troncone, G., and McGee, J.O'D. (1992a). Detection of high risk human papillomavirus in routine cervical smears: strategy for screening. *J. Clin. Pathol.*, **45**, 385–90.

Herrington, C.S., Evans, M.F., Gray, W., McGee, J.O'D., Hallam, N.F., and Charnock, F.M. (1992b). HPV 16 DNA and prediction of high grade CIN. *Lancet*, **339**, 1352–3.

Herrington, C.S., Troncone, G., Evans, M.F., and McGee, J.O'D. (1992c). Screening for high and low risk human papilomavirus types in single routine cervical smears by non-isotopic *in situ* hybridization. *Cytopathology*, **3**, 71–8.

Herrington, C.S., Anderson, S.M., Graham, A.K., and McGee, J.O'D. (1993). The discrimination of high risk HPV types by *in situ* hybridization and the polymerase chain reaction. *Histochem. J.*, **25**, 191–8.

Herrington, C.S., Anderson, S.M., Troncone, G., de Angelis, M.L., Noell, H., Chimera,

J., Van Eyck, S.L., and McGee, J.O'D. (1995a). Comparative analysis of human papillomavirus detection by the polymerase chain reaction and nonisotopic *in situ* hybridization (NISH). *J. Clin. Pathol.*, **48**, 415–19.

Herrington, C.S., Evans, M.F., Hallam, N.F., Charnock, F.M., Gray, W., and McGee, J.O'D. (1995b). HPV analysis in the prediction of high grade CIN in patients with low grade cervical cytological abnormalities. *Br. J. Cancer.*, **71**, 206–9.

Herrington, C.S., Evans, M.F., Gray, W., and McGee, J.O'D. (1995c). Morphological correlation of human papillomavirus infection of matched cervical smears and biopsies from patients with persistent mild cervical cytological abnormalities. *Hum. Pathol.*, **26**, 951–5.

Herrington, C.S., Evans, M.F., Gray, W., Charnock, F.M., and McGee, J.O'D. (1996). HPV testing in patients with low grade cervical cytological abnormalities: a follow-up study. *J. Clin. Pathol.*, **49**, 493–6.

Heryet, A.R., and Gatter, K.C. (1992). Immunocytochemistry for light microscopy. In: *Diagnostic molecular pathology. A practical approach*, Vol. 1, (ed. C.S. Herrington and J.O'D. McGee) pp. 7–46. Oxford University Press, Oxford.

Hopman, A.H.N., Ramaekers, F.C.S., Raap, A.K. *et al.* (1988). *In situ* hybridisation as a tool to study numerical chromosome aberrations in solid bladder tumours. *Histochemistry*, **89**, 307–16.

Hopman, A.H.N., Poddighe, P., Moesker, O., and Ramaekers, F.C.S. (1992). Interphase cytogenetics: an approach to the detection of genetic aberrations in tumours. In: *Diagnostic molecular pathology. A practical approach*, Vol. 1, (ed. C.S. Herrington and J.O'D. McGee), pp. 69–102. Oxford University Press, Oxford.

Hopman, A.H.N. (1995). Probe labelling. In: *Non-isotopic methods in molecular biology. A practical approach*, (ed. E. Levy and C.S. Herrington), pp. 1–24. Oxford University Press, Oxford.

Hsu, S.-M., Raine, L., and Fanger, H. (1981). Use of avidin–biotin–peroxidase complex (ABC) in immunoperoxidase techniques. *J. Histochem. Cytochem.*, **29**, 577–80.

Hsu, S.-M., and Soban, E. (1982). Color modification of diaminobenzidine (DAB) precipitation by metallic ions and its application for double immunohistochemistry. *J. Histochem. Cytochem.*, **30**, 1079–82.

Komminoth, P., Long, A., Ray, R., and Wolfe, H.J. (1992). *In situ* polymerase chain reaction detection of viral DNA, single-copy genes and gene rearrangements in cell suspensions and cytospins. *Diagn. Mol. Pathol.*, **1**, 85–97.

Langer, P.R., Waldrop, A.A., and Ward, D.C. (1981). Enzymatic synthesis of biotin-labeled polynucleotides: novel nucleic acid affinity probes. *Proc. Natl. Acad. Sci. USA*, **78**, 6633–7.

Lorincz, A.T., Temple, G.F., Patterson, J.A., Jenson, A.B., Kurman, R.J., and Lancaster, W.D. (1986). Correlation of cellular atypia and human papillomavirus deoxyribonucleic acid sequences in exfoliated cells of the uterine cervix. *Obstet. Gynaecol.*, **68**, 508–12.

Lorincz, A.T., Reid, R., Jenson, A.B. *et al.* (1992). Human papillomavirus infection of the cervix: relative risk associations of 15 common anogenital types. *Obstet. Gynaecol.* **79**, 328–37.

Melchers, W.J.G., Herbrink, P., Walboomers, J.M.M. *et al.* (1989). Optimisation of human papillomavirus genotype determination in cervical scrapes by a modified filter *in situ* hybridisation test. *J. Clin. Microbiol.*, **27**, 106–10.

Melkert, P.W., Hopman, E., van den Brule, A. *et al.* (1993). Prevalence of HPV in cytomorphologically normal cervical smears, as determined by the polymerase chain reaction, is age-dependent. *Int. J. Cancer.*, **53**, 919–23.

Monji, N., Ali, H., and Castro, A. (1980). Quantification of digoxin by enzyme immunoassay: synthesis for a maleimide derivative of digoxigenin succinate for enzyme coupling. *Experientia*, **36**, 1141–3.

Nederlof, P.M., Robinson, D., Abuknesha, R. *et al*. (1989). Three-color fluorescence *in situ* hybridisation for the simultaneous detection of multople nucleic acid sequences. *Cytometry*, **10**, 20–7.

Nuovo, G.J., Gallery, F., MacConnell, P., and Becker, P. (1991). An improved technique for the *in situ* detection of DNA after PCR. *AM. J. Pathol.*, **139**, 1239–44.

O'Leary, J.J., Browne, G., Bashir, M., Crowley, M., Healy, I., and Lewis, F.A. (1995). Non-isotopic detection of DNA in cells and tissues. In: *Non-isotopic methods in molecular biology. A practical approach*, (ed. E. Levy and C.S. Herrington), pp. 51–83. Oxford University Press, Oxford.

O'Leary, J.J., Kennedy, M.M., McGee, J,O'D. (1997). *In situ* amplification: its application to diagnostic pathology. *Curr. Diagn. Pathol.*, in press.

Pao, C.C., Lai, C.-H., Wu, S.-Y., Young, K.-C., Chang, P.-L., and Soong, Y.-K. (1989). Detection of human papillomaviruses in exfoliated cervicovaginal cells by *in situ* DNA hybridisation analysis. *J. Clin. Microbiol.*, **27**, 168–73.

Pezzella, M., Pezzella, F., Galli, C. *et al*. (1987). *In situ* hybridisation of human immunodeficiency virus (HTLV-III) in cryostat sections of lymph nodes of lymphadenopathy syndrome patients. *J. Med. Virol.*, **22**, 135–42.

Pfister, H., Fuchs, P.G. (1987). In: *Papillomaviruses and human disease*, (ed. K. Syrjanen, L. Gissmann, and L.G. Koss), pp. 1–18. Springer-Verlag, Berlin.

Poerter, H., Quantrill, A.M., and Fleming, K.A. B19 parvovirus infection of myocardial cells. *Lancet*, **i**, 535–6.

Ried, T., Baldini, A., Rand, T.C., and Ward, D.C. (1992). Simultaneous visualization of seven different DNA probes by *in situ* hybridization using combinatorial fluorescence and digital imaging microscopy. *Proc. Natl. Acad. Sci. USA*, **89**, 1388–92.

Schiffman, M.H. (1992). Recent progress in defining the epidemiology of human papillomavirus infection and cervical neoplasia. *J. Natl. Cancer Inst.*, **84**, 394–8.

Schiffman, M.H., Vauer, H.M., Hoover, R.N. *et al*. (1993). Epidemiologic evidence showing that human papillomavirus infection causes most cervical intraepithelial neoplasia. *J. Natl. Cancer Inst.*, **85**, 958–64.

Shibata, D. (1992). The polymerase chain reaction and the molecular genetic analysis of tissue biopsies. In: *Diagnostic molecular pathology. A practical approach*, Vol. 2, (ed. C.S. Herrington and J.O'D. McGee), pp. 85–112. Oxford University Press, Oxford.

Smith, T.W., Butler, V., and Haber, E. (1970). Characterisation of antibodies of high affinity and specifity for the digitialis glycoside digoxin. *Biochemistry*, **9**, 331–7.

Sternberger, L.A., Hardy, P.H., Cuculis, J.J., and Meyer, H.G. (1970). The unlabelled antibody-enzyme method of immunohistochemistry. Preparation and properties of soluble antigen-antibody complex (horseradish peroxidase-antihorseradish peroxidase) and its use in identification of spirochetes. *J. Histochem. Cytochem.*, **18**, 315–33.

Syrjanen, K.J., (1987). Biology of HPV infections and their role in squamous cell carcinogeniesis. *Med. Biol.*, **65**, 21–39.

Syrjanen, S., Partanen, P., Mantyjarvi, R., and Syrjanen K. (1988). Sensitivity of *in situ* hybridisation techniques using biotin and ^{35}S labelled human papillomavirus (HPV) DNA probes. *J. Virol Meth.*, **19**, 225–38.

Syrjanen, S. (1992). Viral gene detection by *in situ* hybridization. In: *Diagnostic molecular pathology. A practical approach*, Vol. 1, (ed. C.S. Herrington and J.O'D. McGee), pp. 103–40. Oxford University Press, Oxford.

Toon, P.G., Arrand, J.R., Wilson, L.P., and Sharp, D.S. (1986). Human papillomavirus infection of the uterine cervix of women without cytological signs of neoplasia. *Br. Med. J.*, **293**, 1261–4.

Troncone, G., Anderson, S.M., Herrington, C.S. *et al.* (1992). Comparative analysis of human papillomavirus detection by dot blot hybridisation and non-itotopic *in situ* hybridisation. *J. Clin. Pathol.*, **45**, 866–70.

Valdes, R., Brown, B.A., and Graves, S.W. (1984). Variable cross-reactivity of digoxin metabolites in digoxin immunoassays. *Am. J. Clin. Pathol.*, **82**, 210–13.

Wagner, D., Ikenberg, H., Boehm, N., and Gissmann, L. (1984). Identification of human papillomavirus in cervical swabs by deoxyribonucleic acid *in situ* hybridisation. *Obstet. Gynaecol.*, **64**, 767–72.

Wagner, L. and Worman, C.P. (1988). Colour-contrast staining of two different lymphocyte sub-populations: a two-colour modification of alkaline phosphatase monoclonal anti-alkaline phosphatase complex technique. *Stain Technol.*, **63**, 129–35.

Walboomers, J.M.M., Melkert, P.W.J., van den Brule, A.J., Snijders, P.J.F., and Meijer, C.J.L.M. (1992). The polymerase chain reaction for human papillomavirus screening in diagnostic cytopathology of the cervix. In: *Diagnostic molecular pathology. A practical approach*, Vol. 2, (ed. C.S. Herrington and J.O'D. McGee), pp. 153–71. Oxford University Press, Oxford.

Wells, M., Griffiths, S., Lewis, F., and Bird, C.C. (1987). Demonstration of human papillomavirus types in paraffin processed tissue from human anogenital lesions by *in situ* DNA hybridisation. *J. Pathol.*, **152**, 77–82.

Wolber, R.A. and Lloyd, R.V. (1988). Cytomegalovirus detection by nonisotopic *in situ* DNA hybridisation and viral antigen immunostaining using a two-colour technique. *Hum. Pathol.*, **19**, 736–41.

Zhou, X.G., Hamilton-Dutoit, S.H., Yan, Q.H., Pallesen, G. (1994). High frequency of Epstein–Barr virus in Chinese peripheral T-cell lymphoma. *Histopathology*, **24**, 115–22.

Appendix 8.1

Materials

All organic chemicals, unless otherwise stated, were purchased from BDH (UK).

1. Digoxigenin dUTP and alkaline phosphatase conjugated anti-digoxigenin (Boehringer Mannheim, Germany; from kit no. 1093 657)

2. Biotin-7-dATP and dNTP mixture for biotinylation (Gibco/BRL)

3. DNase 1 (Worthingtons, UK; Cat. No. L500 06330)

4. DNA polymerase 1 (Boerhinger Mannheim, Germany; Cat. No. 642 711)

5. Glycogen (Boerhinger Mannheim, Germany; Cat. No. 901 393)

6. Tris–EDTA (TE)—10 mM Tris–HCl, 1 mM EDTA, pH 8.

7. Four-spot multiwell slides (Hendley, Essex: spot diameter 12 mm)

8. Decon 90 (Philip Harris, UK; Cat. No. D35-460)

9. Aminopropyltriethoxysilane (Sigma, UK; Cat. No. A3648)

10. Proteinase K (Boerhinger Mannheim, Germany; Cat. No. 745 723)

11. Phosphate buffered saline (PBS)—10 mM phosphate, 150 mM naCl, pH 7.4

12, Methanol–acetic acid (3:1, v/v)

13. 4% (w/v) paraformaldehyde (BDH, UK) in PBS—dissolve 4 g of paraformaldehyde in each 100 ml of PBS by heating.

14. Hydrogen peroxide (BDH, UK).

15. Formamide (Sigma, UK; Cat. No. F7503)

16. Dextran sulfate (Sigma, UK; Cat. No. D6001)

17. Saline sodium citrate (SSC)—1 × SSC: 150 mM NaCl, 15 mM sodium citrate

18. Coverslips (Chance, Raymond Lamb, UK; Cat. No. E/23—22 × 64 mm, 22 × 50 mm, and 14 mm)

19. Terasaki plates (Gibco/Nunc, UK; Cat. No. 1-36528A)

20. Tris-buffered saline (TBS)—50 mM Tris–HCl, 100 mM NaCl pH 7.2

21. Bovine serum albumin (BSA) (Sigma, UK; Cat. No. B2518)

22. Triton 100 (Sigma, UK; Cat. No. T8761)

23. Streptavidin–peroxidase (Dako, UK; Cat. No. P397)

24. Avidin alkaline phosphatase (Dako, UK, Cat. No. D365)

25. Monoclonal anti-digoxin (Sigma)

26. Monoclonal anti-biotin (Dako, UK, Cat. No. M743)

27. Biotinylated rabbit anti-mouse [F(ab') fragment] (Dako, UK, Cat. No. E413)

28. Substrate buffer—50 mM Tris–HCl, 100 mM NaCl, 1 mM $MgCl_2$, pH 9.5.

29. 3-Amino-9-ethylcarbazole (Sigma, UK, Cat. No. A5754)

30. Nitroblue tetrazolium (NBT) (Sigma, UK, Cat. No. N6876)

31. 5-Bromo-4-chloro-3-indolylphosphate (BCIP) (Sigma, UK, Cat. No. B8503)

Methods

Probe labelling

1. Mix:

	Digoxigenin	Biotin
Plasmid DNA	1 μg	1 μg
Nucleotide mix*	1 μl	5 μl
Biotin-dATP	–	2.5 μl
DNase 1[†]	1–5 ng	1–5 ng

*For biotin labelling, the nucleotide mix contains 0.2 mM of each of dCTP, dTTP, and dGTP. This is made up from individual nucleotides. For digoxigenin labelling, the mix contains all nucleotides including digoxigenin-dUTP/dTTP at a concentration of 1 mM.
[†]The amount of DNase required is assessed by alkaline gel electrophoresis followed by Southern transfer and enzymatic detection. DNase is adjusted to give a median probe size of 200–400 bp.

2. Add distilled water (dH$_2$O) to 49 μl and incubate at 37 °C for 2 min.
3. Add 1 μl DNA polymerase 1(5 U/μl) and incubate at 14 °C for 150 min.
4. Add 5 μl 200 mM EDTA and heat at 75 °C for 10 min to terminate reaction.
5. Add 1 μl glycogen (20 mg/ml).
6. Add 1/10th vol 3 M NaOAc, pH 6, then 2 vols absolute EtOH.
7. Incubate on dry ice for 20 min or at −20°C overnight.
8. Spin at 12 000 rpm for 20 min.
9. Wash in 80% ethanol (EtOH) × 4.
10. Lyophilize and resuspend in 50 μl TE.
11. Store labelled probes at either −20 or 4 °C. If stored at −20 °C, do not repeatedly freeze–thaw.

This procedure can be scaled up by multiplication of the reaction volumes.

Preparation of slides

1. Clean four-spot multiwell slides (12 mm spot diameter) in 2% Decon 90 at 60 °C for 30 min.
2. Rinse in dH$_2$O then acetone, and air dry.
3. Immerse in 2% aminopropylethoxysilane in acetone for 30 min.
4. Wash in dH$_2$O and air dry at 37 °C.
5. Slides prepared in this way can be stored indefinitely at room temperature.

Preparation of biopsies

Dewaxing of sections

1. Cut 5 μm sections from routine paraffin-embedded blocks on to slides prepared as above.

146

2. Bake sections either (i) overnight at 60°C or (ii) for 45 min at 75°C.
3. Store slides at room temperature.
4. When required, heat to 75°C for 15 min.
5. Plunge into xylene and wash for 10 min. Change xylene once.
6. Clear in 99% ethanol (industrial grade).
7. Wash in dH_2O.

Unmasking of nucleic acids
1. Store proteinase K at 20 mg/ml in dH_2O at −20°C.
2. Dilute to 500 μg/ml in PBS.
3. Spot on to slides, place in Terasaki plates, and float in water bath at 37°C for 15 min.
4. Wash in dH_2O and air dry at 75°C.

Alternatively, pepsin-HCl can be used (see Chapter 7 and Hopman *et al.* 1992)

Preparation of cervical smears
1. Use smears fixed routinely in 70% ethanol.
2. Fix in fresh methanol–acetic acid (3:1; v/v) pre-equilibrated to −20°C for 10 min.
3. Fix in 4% (w/v) paraformaldehyde in PBS for 15 min at room temperature.
4. Wash in PBS containing 0.2% (w/v) glycine and then PBs for 5 min each at room temperature.
5. Block endogenous peroxidase activity by incubation in 0.1% (w/v) sodium azide containing 0.3% hydrogen peroxide for 20 min at room temperature.
6. Wash in PBS then incubate in proteinase K (1 μg/ml in PBS) for 15 min at 37°C.
7. Wash in PBS for 5 min at room temperature then post-fix in 4% (w/v) paraformaldehyde for 5 min at room temperature.
8. Wash in PBS/glycine then PBS for 5 min each and air-dry.

Application of probe to section
For each spot:
1. Add 10 μl (200 ng) of each of biotin- and/or digoxigenin-labelled probes to each 70 μl of HM.
2. Add TE to make 100 μl total volume.

3. Spot 8 μl of the mixture on to each well for biopsies and 50 μl to each cervical smear.

4. Cover each spot on a multiwell slide with a 14 mm round coverslip, or each cervical smear with a 22 × mm coverslip. These need not be silanized and should not be sealed with rubber solution as is frequently recommended.

Denaturation/hybridization
1. Place slides in Terasaki plates (2 slides/plate).
2. Denature on a hot plate in hot air oven at 95 °C for 15 min.
3. Hybridize at 42 °C in hot air oven for 2 h.

Stringency washing and blocking procedure
1. Wash slides in 4 × SSC at room temperature, twice (5 min each).
2. Wash in appropriate solution for high stringency, e.g. 50% formamide/0.1 × SSC (if required for discriminating closely homologous sequences).
3. Wash in 4 × SSC at room temperature for 5 min.
4. Incubate for 30 min in blocking solution (TBT)—TBS containing 5% (w/v) bovine serum albumin, 0.05% (v/v) Triton 100.

Adjust all washing solutions to pH 7 with 5 M HCl. The temperature of the solution should be monitored *directly* using a mercury thermometer. Washing should be carried out for 30 min (see Herrington *et al.* 1990, 1993; Herrington and McGee, 1994).

Routine detection of digoxigenin-labelled probes
1. Incubate at room temperature for 30 minutes in monoclonal anti-digoxin (Sigma, UK) diluted 1:10 000 in TBT.
2. Wash in TBS for 5 min, twice.
3. Incubate at room temperature for 30 min in biotinylated rabbit anti-mouse [F(ab′)$_2$ fragment] diluted 1:200 in TBT.
4. Wash in TBS for 5 min, twice.
5. Incubate in avidin peroxidase diluted 1:75 in TBT containing 5% non-fat milk.
6. Remove unbound conjugate by washing twice in TBS for 5 min.
7. Incubate in the peroxidase substrate, 3-amino-9-ethylcarbazole (AEC)/ H_2O_2, for 30 min at room temperature.
8. Terminate the reaction by washing in distilled water for 5 min.
9. Air dry the slides at 42 °C and mount in glycerol jelly.

Double probe detection

1. Incubate at room temperature for 30 min in a mixture of streptavidin–peroxidase conjugate, diluted 1:100 in TBT, and alkaline phosphatase-conjugated anti-digoxigenin, diluted 1:600 in TBT; in practice 1 μl of antibody and 6 μl of streptavidin is added to 600 μl of TBT.
2. Remove unbound conjugate by washing twice in 50 mM Tris–HCl, 100 mM NaCl pH7.2 (TBS) for 5 min.
3. Incubate in the peroxidase substrate, 3-amino-9-ethylcarbazole (AEC), for 30 min at room temperature.
4. Terminate the reaction by thorough washing in TBS.
5. Wash in substrate buffer for 5 min at room temperature.
6. Incubate in NBT/BCIP for 20–40 min.
7. Terminate the reaction by washing in distilled water for 5 min.
8. Air cry the slides at 42 °C and mount in glycerol jelly.

Amplified dual detection

1. Incubate at room temperature for 30 min in monoclonal anti-biotin diluted 1:50 in TBT.
2. Wash in TBS for 5 min, twice.
3. Incubate at room temperature for 30 min in biotinylated rabbit anti-mouse [F(ab')$_2$ fragment] diluted 1:200 in TBT.
4. Wash in TBS for 5 min, twice.
5. Continue from step 1 of the dual detection protocol.

Substrate preparation

Many substrates can now be purchased in tablet form (e.g. Sigma, UK).

NBT/BCIP

1. Dissolve 10 mg NBT in 200 μl dimethylformamide (DMF).
2. Add 1 ml substrate buffer at 37 °C and add mixture dropwise to 30 ml substrate buffer at 37 °C.
3. Dissolve 5 mg BCIP in 200 μl DMF and add slowly to the above mixture.
4. Aliquot and store at −20 °C.

AEC

1. Dissolve 2 mg of AEC in 1.2 ml dimethylsulfoxide in a glass tube.
2. Add to 10 ml 20 mM acetate buffer pH 5.0–5.2.
3. Add 0.8 μl of 30% (v/v) hydrogen peroxide and use the final mix immediately.

Glycerol jelly (Bancroft and Stevens 1977)

1. Dissolve 10 g gelatine in 60 ml dH$_2$O in 37 °C water bath.
2. Add 70 ml glycerol and 0.25 g phenol.
3. Store at room temperature (solid) or in 42 °C oven (liquid).

9

Combined *in situ* hybridization and immunocytochemistry; investigation of viral pathogenesis at the light and electron microscope levels

KENNETH A. FLEMING and ADRIENNE L. MOREY

Introduction

Simple detection of viral nucleic acid by *in situ* hybridization (ISH) has been practised for many years (Brahic and Haase 1978). While this is of considerable value in allowing, for example, estimation of the prevalence of various viruses in different diseases (Myerson *et al.* 1984), it has certain limitations. Not infrequently, it is impossible to identify unequivocally the type and range of cells infected, for example, virus may be present in mononuclear cells in a tissue or organ, but whether these are macrophages, lymphocytes, endothelial cells, etc. can be impossible to determine. Even when viral nucleic acid is present in cells in an epithelium, it may not necessarily be present in an epithelial cell, e.g. it may be in an infiltrating inflammatory cell or Langheran's cell. This problem of precise identification of the infected cell type is particularly acute when radioisotopes are used and the resolution of the ISH signal is frequently poor. A second limitation of simple ISH is that it is not possible to determine which, if any, viral proteins are being synthesized at the time of biopsy and thus to correlate the presence of that protein with particular pathological features. It is important to note in this context that detection of mRNA for a protein does not necessarily equate with synthesis of that protein. The third limitation of simple ISH is that it only permits limited analysis of any associated pathological process. Thus, while polymorphs can be identified with some certainty, the correct assignment of associated mononuclear inflammatory cells as macrophages or lymphocytes may be impossible. Furthermore, subdivision of infiltrating lymphocytes into B or T cells, CD4$^+$, or CD8$^+$ cells, and detection of expression of activation markers (e.g. CD25), cytokines, integrins, HLA molecules, etc. by the inflammatory or parenchymal cells, cannot be achieved. Increasingly, information of this sort is required to provide insight into the pathobiology of viral infections.

One way of overcoming the above limitations is to combine ISH for viral nucleic acid with immunocytochemistry (ICC) for viral or cellular proteins. An increasing range of monoclonal and polyclonal antibodies to a wide range of cell lineage-specific molecules, activation markers, cytokines, and viral proteins should facilitate such studies. While performance of ISH and ICC on consecutive sections or replicates of tissue culture cells can give some of this information, there is always some doubt about the accuracy of these investigations, particularly where only occasional cells are infected by the virus. Accordingly, combined ISH and ICC on the same tissue section or cell preparation is the most accurate method of investigating questions concerning the nature of the infected cells and the presence of certain viral proteins. Despite this, relatively few such investigations have been published (see below) and the analysis of host response and its relationship to viral gene expression has barely been initiated. This slow start probably reflects the view that the technology is very difficult and capricious. However, this view is incorrect, as will be described below.

The first section of this chapter will discuss aspects of the technology required to perform combined ISH and ICC at the light microscope (LM) level and provide some illustrative applications. The second section will similarly detail the approach used for ultrastructural ISH including combined ISH/ICC.

Combined ISH/ICC at the light microscope level

Technical aspects

General considerations

The aim of the procedure is to localize nucleic acid and antigen at the same time in the same tissue or cellular preparation. This is done by performing ISH and ICC sequentially. In general, the order in which ICC/ISH is performed is determined by the need to preserve antigenicity. The high temperatures and/or strong alkalai used to denature nucleic acid targets can also denature antigen, leading to loss of antigenicity. Accordingly, if ISH is performed first, then subsequent ICC may be unsuccessful. A lower temperature denaturation with added formamide may be tried, but again, the effects on antigenicity must be checked. While certain antigens are sufficiently robust to withstand the ISH procedure, performing ICC before ISH generally results in better signal for the ICC. Therefore, our practice is to perform the ICC procedure first, followed by ISH. Only if this fails, is the order reversed. With antigens that require protease digestion (trypsin, etc.) for detection in formalin-fixed material, the digestion step usually does not need to be repeated for the ISH.

A fundamental consideration when determining the optimal combination of ICC and ISH signals is whether to use isotopic ISH. In theory, where nucleic acid and antigenic targets are completely coincident, the combination of isotopic ISH with ICC should be ideal (see Chapter 4). Thus, performance of isotopic ISH first would allow detection of ISH signal, even though it was 'buried' beneath the subsequent ICC signal. The major disadvantage of isotopic ISH is the poor signal resolution. This, and other disadvantages (prolonged development time, inability to control the development process, safety hazards, and cost), has meant that although isotopic ISH has been successfully used in a number of combined ISH/ICC investigations (Blum *et al.* 1984; Brahic *et al.* 1984; Gendelman *et al.* 1985; Yoshioka *et al.* 1992; Gosztonyi *et al.* 1994), non-isotopic ISH is generally the preferred option. We generally prefer to use digoxigenin rather than biotin as the non-isotopic probe label in order to avoid artefacts caused by the presence of endogeneous biotin.

Antigen preservation/access

Several factors affect antigenic preservation and/or access. Of these, the most important is fixation. The optimum fixatives for ISH appear to be either organic solvents, such as alcohols and acetone (with or without chloroform and acid), or aldehyde fixatives, such as formaldehyde (Mullink *et al.* 1989). Unfortunately, many antigens are rendered 'inaccessible' or denatured by cross-linking fixatives such as formaldehyde. To overcome this problem, frozen sections can be used (with or without fixation in a precipitant such as alcohol), although the harshness of the ISH procedure may cause the fragile frozen sections to fragment. However, successful ISH/ICC on frozen sections has been reported and this may be the only available approach when the antigenic target cannot survive aldehyde fixation (Mullink *et al.* 1989; van der Loos *et al.* 1989).

Aldehyde fixation has particular advantages in preserving morphology and is used where at all possible. Many antigens that are masked by formalin fixation can be rendered accessible by protease digestion or other antigen retrieval techniques. Protease digestion is particularly suitable for combined ISH/ICC, since the protease digestion can fulfil two functions; it not only 'unmasks' the antigen for ICC, but also allows efficient access to nucleic acid for subsequent ISH. While a variety of proteolytic enzymes can be used (see Table 9.1), we have found that protease VIII (Sigma) permits determination of the optimal conditions most easily. Conversely, some antigens are digested by protease (Graham *et al.* 1991), making it necessary to perform ICC first, with subsequent ISH incorporating a protease step. It is advisable to pre-incubate protease solutions prior to application to sections in order to autodigest any nucleases present.

Nucleic acid preservation/access

In general, nucleic acid preservation is not a particular problem in combined ISH/ICC. However, it is necessary to ensure that all the reagents used in both

Table 9.1 Proteolytic enzymes for combined ISH/ICC

Enzyme	Advantages and disadvantages
Proteinase K	Efficient; sometimes leaves non-specific nucleolar staining
Proteinase VIII	Gentle, effective; wide optimum concentration range
Pronase	Rather unstable
Pepsin/HCl	Effective; must carefully control concentration of both pepsin and HCl

ISH/ICC are nuclease free, and in particular RNase free. It is theoretically possible that certain sera used for ICC contain RNases that digest RNA targets. This problem can be overcome by either purifying the antibody, using a different antiserum, adding diethylpyrocarbonate to the serum (Yoshioka *et al.* 1992), or performing the ICC after the ISH procedure if the antigen is sufficiently robust. It should be noted that access to nucleic acids may be partially restricted by the presence of chromogenic substrate from a preceding ICC procedure, resulting in a slight reduction in the ISH signal (van der Loos *et al.* 1989; Porter *et al.* 1990). The magnitude of this effect is likely to depend on the relative spatial locations of the antigenic and nucleic acid targets.

Signal contrast/differentiation

Given that a non-isotopic ISH protocol is used, a second important factor determining the success of combined ISH/ICC is the choice of contrasting detection signals. Ideally, one should use a detection system for both the ISH and ICC procedures that is optimally sensitive and specific. A variety of enzymatic detection systems are available with reaction products that which will survive any subsequent ISH or ICC procedure (see Table 9.2).

Table 9.2 Signal combinations used in ISH/ICC

Enzyme	Substrate	Colour	Advantages
Alkaline phosphatase	NBT/BCIP	Blue/black	Optimum; highest sensitivity good resolution, and resistant to subsequent procedures
	Fast Red/naphthol-AS-MX PO$_4$	Red	Reasonably sensitive, but less so than NBT/BCIP. Reasonably good resolution
	New fuchsin/naphthol-AS-BI PO4	Crimson	" "
Peroxidase	DAB	Brown	Excellent resolution, rapid, but poor contrast with blue and relatively low sensitivity. Resistant to subsequent procedures
	Aminoethylcarbazole	Red/orange	Excellent resolution but tends to be dissolved by alcohol

N.B. The reaction conditions for the substrates arre as described in standard textbooks.

Alkaline phosphatase with nitroblue tetrazolium/5-bromo-3-chloro-4-indolyl phosphate (NBT/BCIP) is generally acknowledged to be the most sensitive and specific, producing a blue/black signal. The use of alkaline phosphatase with New Fuchsin or Fast Red substrates (which are slightly less sensitive than NBT/BCIP) produces a red product. The combination of these two detection systems (usually red for ICC and blue/black for ISH) gives optimal colour contrast, sensitivity, and specificity. If ICC is performed first, subsequent manipulations in the ISH procedure should destroy any residual alkaline phosphatase, thus a second alkaline phosphatase detection system may be used to visualize the ISH signal without false-positive reactions. Circumstances requiring less than optimal sensitivity allow use of the other detection systems listed in Table 9.2, of which peroxidase with AEC is particularly useful for either ICC or ISH.

Antibodies labelled with colloidal gold provide an additional possibility for signal detection; use of colloidal gold (usually with silver enhancement) in either of the procedures gives good contrast with a red signal, but in combination with blue/black is more difficult to discriminate.

While, in theory, it should be possible to use colour reactions for ICC and non-isotopic ISH that produce a third colour when signals are completely coincident, in practice, this has proved extremely difficult (van der Loos *et al.* 1989), if not impossible (personal observations), to achieve. One way around the problem of coincident signal is to use confocal microscopy and digital image processing; for example, colloidal gold signal from one target, detected under reflected light, could be digitally combined with fluorescent signal from the second target and a composite image created. Alternatively, two different fluorescent labels could be used (Somasundaran *et al.* 1994). The obvious disadvantage of the use of fluorescent labels, however, is the impermanent nature of the labelling.

A simple protocol for combined ICC/non-isotopic ISH for a DNA target in paraffin-embedded tissue using contrasting chromogenic substrates is shown in the Appendix [see also Morey and Fleming (1992) and Moray *et al.* (1992) for additional details).

Applications of combined ICC/ISH at the LM level
Identification of infected cell type
As mentioned at the beginning of the chapter, identification of cells containing viral nucleic acid can often be problematic in simple ISH. However, the range of cellular tropism of a virus is a fundamental question in understanding its pathobiology. Indeed, recognition of unexpected tropism has been one of the particularly useful outcomes of combined ISH/ICC. We have used this approach to examine the range of cell types containing human parvovirus B19 (Porter *et al.* 1990; Morey and Fleming 1992; Morey *et al.* 1992). This is a common and usually trivial infection in childhood. However, when a non-

immune, pregnant woman is infected, the virus can also infect the fetus, causing intrauterine death with cardiac failure. Combined ICC/ISH studies on infected fetal tissues revealed B19 nucleic acid within nucleated red cells, macrophages, and occasional myocardial cells (Porter *et al.* 1990; Morey *et al.* 1992). Although replication in myocardial cells is unlikely, given B19's strict tropism for a subgroup of late erythroid precursor cells *in vitro* (Morey and Fleming 1992), it is possible that immune-mediated damage induced by the presence of virus in the myocardium could contribute to fetal morbidity.

Investigation of the range of cell types involved in Epstein–Barr virus-associated lymphomas has been another important application of combined ICC/ISH studies. In Hodgkin's disease, for example, EBV nucleic acid has been found not only in CD30-positive Reed–Sternberg cells and their mononuclear variants, but also in smaller, peanut agglutinin-positive cells, which were negative for T, B, and macrophage markers (Jiwa *et al.* 1993), suggesting downregulation of cell lineage markers by the virus. Analysis of cases of lymphomatoid granulomatosis of the lung (Guinee *et al.* 1994) has confirmed that, in the majority of cases, the disease represents a monoclonal proliferation of EBV-infected B cells with a prominent reactive T cell component, rather than an angiocentric T cell lymphoma, as previously thought.

Analogous investigations have been performed on brain tissue from patients with several virus-associated conditions, including progressive multifocal leukoencephalopathy. Light microscopy (LM) had previously indicated that oligodendrocytes were the cells infected by JC papovavirus in this condition. However, initial ISH experiments had suggested that a wider range of cells, namely astrocytes, neurones, and endothelial cells, were also involved. Use of combined ISH/ICC showed that both oligodendrocytes and occasional bizarre astrocytes (glial fibrillary acid protein-positive cells) were infected, but that there was no evidence of endothelial or neuronal involvement (Ironside *et al.* 1989). In subacute sclerosing panencephalitis (SSPE), the relationship between the measles virus genome and neurofibrillary tangles was analysed by combining ISH for measles virus nucleic acid and ICC for tau-2 protein (McQuaid *et al.* 1994). The results in several cases of long-standing SSPE clearly showed that measles virus was co-localized with tau-2-positive neurofibrils. These data suggested that neurofibrillary tangle formation can occur as a result of viral infection, a finding that may have implications for Alzheimer's disease.

In encephalitis due to human immunodeficiency virus (HIV), combined ISH/ICC has shown HIV nucleic acid and protein to be present almost exclusively within brain macrophages (Gosztonyi *et al.* 1994). Combined studies have also shown that HIV-containing cerebral macrophages co-express ferritin, a marker of activation (Yoshioka *et al.* 1992). Studies on the cellular localization of cytomegalovirus in HIV-positive patients have confirmed that virus is present not only in epithelial cells, as light microscopy had shown, but also in endothelial cells (Roberts *et al.* 1989); up to 60% of CMV-positive (cytomegalovirus) cells in the gut of immunosuppressed individuals were positive for factor VIII, suggesting that CMV infection, in this situation at least, is primarily vasculitic.

Correlation of viral presence with mRNA expression, protein synthesis, and pathogenicity

Combined ISH/ICC has also been used to examine the relationship between the presence of viral nucleic acid in a cell, expression of particular genes, and the pathogenicity of the virus. This approach addresses the question; which genes in a virus are responsible for particular aspects of its pathogenicity, especially cytolysis? an example of this has been the investigation of Semliki Forest virus infection of the CNS (central nervous system) in mice (Balluz *et al.* 1993). BALB/c mice were innoculated intranasally with either virulent (SFV4) or avirulent (A7) strains of the virus and combined ISH/ICC was used to analyse which cells became infected and how cytolysis related to viral gene expression. The results showed that both strains of virus infected the same types of cells (neurones and oligodendrocytes) but that only the lethal strain (SFV4) showed virus-specific antigen in the damaged cells. In this situation, it appears that viral gene expression is causing cytopathic effects.

In other viral infections, a host immune-mediated response to viral antigen appears to be the cause of cell damage, rather than direct viral cytopathy. In such situations, downregulation of gene expression may lead to viral persistence. For example, early work on Theiler's encephalomyelitis virus (a persistent, demyelinating disease of murine CNS) showed that, in inflamed areas, many cells contained viral genome, but far fewer contained viral antigen (Brahic *et al.* 1984). It was suggested that viral persistence in the face of a brisk immune response may be explained by the fact that a proportion of the infected cells did not express viral antigens and therefore were not destroyed by the host immune response.

Hepatitis B virus infection of the liver is another disease where viral persistence may result from downregulation of gene expression. Combined ISH/ICC with both radiolabelled (Blum *et al.* 1984) and digoxigenin-labelled probes (Lau *et al.* 1991) has been used to analyse the cellular relationship between viral replication and expression of surface and core antigens in this disease. These investigations have shown that core antigen was not found in cells with high levels of viral replication and that, conversely, core antigen was present when viral replication was low. Viral replication was also not present in cells containing surface antigen. Accordingly, as in Theiler's encephalomyelitis virus, the absence of protein antigens thought to be the target of viral immune surveillance suggests a mechanism by which viral persistence may occur.

Ultrastructural ISH for localization of viruses

Introduction

Despite recent advances in understanding the molecular biology of certain viruses, relatively little work has been done on the morphological and topographic aspects of viral intracellular nucleic acid metabolism. The extension of ISH techniques to the ultrastructural level provides a means of exploring this area. Early attempts at ultrastructural viral localization using radiolabelled probes and autoradiographic detection were complicated by poor spatial resolution of signal and long processing times (Croissant *et al.* 1972; Geuskens and May, 1974). It is only relatively recently, with the development of efficient non-isotopic probe labelling strategies and immunogold detection methods, that the technique has begun to achieve its potential. Non-isotopic probes have been used to localize both DNA and RNA viruses at the ultrastructural level in infected tissues and cell cultures. Studies have been performed on plant viruses as well as animal viruses, using a variety of different probe types, and hybridization methodologies.

Table 9.3 Ultrastructural viral *in situ* hybridization

Virus	Target	Method	Reference
DNA viruses			
CMV	DNA	Pre-embedding DNA probe/biotin	Wolber *et al.* 1988
	DNA	Post-embedding DNA probe/digoxigenin	Cennachi *et al.* 1993
HSV-I	RNA	Pre-embedding DNA probe/biotin	Wolber *et al.* 1989
	DNA	Post-embedding DNA probe/biotin	Puvion-Dutilleul and Puvion 1989 Puvion-Dutilleul *et al.* 1989
	DNA/RNA	Post-embedding DNA probe/biotin	Puvion-Dutilleul and Puvion 1991a
	RNA	Post-embedding DNA probe/biotin	Besse *et al.* 1995
Adenovirus-5	DNA	Post-embedding DNA probe/biotin	Puvion-Dutilleul and Puvion 1990a Puvion-Dutilleul and Puvion 1990b Puvion-Dutilleul and Pichard 1993 Besse and Puvion-Dutilleul 1994
	DNA/RNA	Post-embedding DNA probe/biotin Post-embedding DNA probe/biotin	Puvion-Dutilleul and Puvion 1991b Puvion-Dutilleul *et al.* 1992
	DNA (ds and ss)	Post-embedding DNA probe/biotin	Puvion-Dutilleul and Pichard 1992
	DNA	post-embedding and whole mount DNA probe/biotin	Jiao *et al.* 1992
HPV	DNA (types 6/11)	Pre-embedding DNA probe/biotin	Tsutsumi *et al.* 1991

An overview of the publications to date is provided in Table 9.3. Ultrastructural non-isotopic ISH permits unequivocal identification and exact spatial localization of nucleic acid targets, allowing examination of the intracellular location of viral nucleic acids at different stages of the infective cycle, as well as the relationship between viral replication and cytopathic effects. The ease with which non-isotopic *in situ* detection of viral nucleic acid can be combined with immunohistochemical labelling of viral proteins makes the technique an especially powerful one. For example, we have combined ISH for parvovirus B19 DNA with immunocytochemical labelling of B19 capsid and non-structural proteins (Morey *et al.* 1993, 1995). The protocols we have employed are detailed in the appendix and a discussion of various methodological issues is given below.

Table 9.3 Continued

Virus	Target	Method	Reference
	DNA (types 6b)	Pre-embedding DNA probe/biotin	Yun and Sherwood 1992
	DNA (types 6/11, 16/18)	Post embedding DNA probes/HRP (horseradish peroxidase)	Multhaupt *et al.* 1992
	DNA (type 2a)	Post-embedding DNA probe/biotin	Hagari *et al.* 1993
Parvovirus B19	DNA	Post-embedding DNA probe/digoxigenin	Morey *et al.* 1993
	DNA (+protein)	Post-embedding DNA probe/digoxigenin	Morey *et al.* 1995
EBV	DNA	Post-embedding and cryosections DNA probe/biotin	Mandry *et al.* 1993
RNA viruses			
HIV-I	RNA	Post-embedding DNA probe/biotin	Fournier *et al.* 1991
	RNA (+protein)	Post-embedding DNA probe/biotin	Escaig-Haye *et al.* 1992
	RNA	Post-embedding DNA probe/biotin	Baccetti *et al.* 1994
	RNA	Pre- and post-embedding DNA probe/biotin	Somasundaran *et al.* 1994
Poliovirus	RNA	Post-embedding DNA and RNA probes/biotin	Troxler *et al.* 1990
	RNA (2 regions, + protein	Post-embedding RNA probes/biotin and digoxigenin	Troxler *et al.* 1992 Egger *et al.* 1994
	RNA	Cell fraction mount RNA probe/biotin	Bienz *et al.* 1992
Bamboo mosaic virus	RNA	Post-embedding RNA probe/digoxigenin	Lin *et al.* 1993

Technical considerations

Hybridization methods

Successful detection of nucleic acid sequences at the ultrastructural level is a compromise between the necessity of maintaining acceptable morphology while affording sufficient access for hybridization. Ultrastructural ISH studies basically fall into four categories depending on the methodology employed.

1. *Pre-embedding hybridization*, involving hybridization to cells or tissues permeabilized with detergent and/or proteolytic agents; after the hybridization procedure the material is osmicated, embedded in plastic, and thin-sectioned.
2. *Post-embedding hybridization*, involving hybridization to thin sections of cells or tissues embedded in hydrophilic acrylic resins, such as Lowicryl K4M and LR White.
3. *Hybridization to ultrathin frozen sections*.
4. *Hybridization to whole mount cells*.

The first reports of ultrastructural localization of viral sequences by non-isotopic ISH employed a pre-embedding hybridization method using fibroblasts infected with CMV and HSV-1 (Wolber *et al.* 1988, 1989). Morphological preservation was fairly poor, and the majority of subsequent studies have employed post-embedding techniques. There is currently only one report of the use of ultrathin cryosections for viral localization (Mandry *et al.* 1993), as well as a single study employing a 'whole mount' approach (Jiao *et al* 1992). Each technique has different advantages and disadvantages, which are summarized in Table 9.4.

Pre-embedding protocols require permeabilization treatment prior to hybridization. This can result in loss of cellular constituents and necessarily causes some morphological deterioration. Pre-embedding hybridization should theoretically provide reasonably good sensitivity as it permits detection of

Table 9.4 Comparison of hybridization methods

Method	Advantages	Disadvantages
Pre-embedding	Reasonable sensitivity	Immediate processing required; loss of cellular constituents; variable probe penetration; poor penetration of gold colloids; poor resolution of DAB signal
Post-embedding	Reasonable morphology; storage possible	Relative insensitivity (surface hybridization)
Ultrathin frozen	Greatest sensitivity; rapidity; storage possible	Poor morphology; infection risk
Whole mount	Signal throughout cell	Loss of cellular constituents; poor morphology

target located anywhere within the cell. However, lack of signal over a particular cellular structure may reflect either true absence of target, or lack of penetration of reagents owing to insufficient or uneven permeabilization (Wolber *et al.* 1988. 1989). This is particularly a problem for colloidal gold–antibody conjugates because of their large size. Some groups have chosen to use antibody–peroxidase conjugates and electron-dense DAB substrate as an alternative method of probe visualization (Tsutsumi *et al.* 1991; Yun and Sherwood, 1992); however, this produces a poor resolution signal which cannot be quantitated.

Post-embedding techniques involve application of probes to material embedded in a variety of hydrophilic, acrylic resins. These resins were developed for ultrastructural immunocytochemistry, but are also ideally suited to ISH, since resin sections can withstand enzymatic digestions, denaturation, and incubation in formamide. Resins that have been used in viral ISH studies include Lowicryl K4M (Puvion-Dutilleul and Puvion, 1989), Lowicryl HM20 (Lin *et al.* 1993), LR White (Troxler *et al.* 1990), LR Gold (Troxler *et al.* 1992) and Bioacryl (Cennachi *et al.* 1993). Although Lowicryl K4M has been the most widely used resin, the embedding process is rather laborious and newer resins that are easier to handle are becoming more popular. The various resins appear to provide similar sensitivity (Troxler *et al.* 1990; Cennachi *et al.* 1993; Morey *et al.* 1993), although Bioacryl has been reported to preserve ultrastructure better than Lowicryl K4M (Cenacchi *et al.* 1993). Hybridization to nucleic acid targets in sections of resin-embedded material can only occur at the surface of the section. For that reason, the technique is suitable only for the detection of high copy sequences concentrated at very well-defined sites. Since productively infected cells generally contain large numbers of viral genomes, the relative insensitivity of the post-embedding approach is not usually a problem, although the method would not be recommended for localization of viral sequences in latently infected cells.

Comparative studies have shown hybridization to ultrathin cryosections to be the most sensitive method of ultrastucutal hybridization (Dirks *et al.* 1992). However, morphology is poor (Mandry *et al.* 1993) and there are safety hazards associated with sectioning unfixed infected tissues; thus, the use of ultrathin cryosections has not been widely adopted for viral studies.

In preliminary experiments we found that pre-embedding hybridization produced unacceptable morphological damage and that a post-embedding protocol employing LR White resin (see EM Protocol 1) provided a reasonable compromise between the demands for morphological preservation and sensitivity.

Fixation

Aldehyde fixation of tissues is required for all ultrastructural hybridization methods (except where 'freeze-substitution' embedding is performed). High concentrations of glutaraldehyde impair denaturation and detection of double-stranded DNA (Puvion-Dutilleul and Puvion, 1991a); however, the use of paraformaldehyde alone does not provide sufficiently good morphological preservation. The addition of a low concentration (<0.5%) of glutaraldehyde to freshly prepared paraformaldehyde (2–4%) appears to help preserve morphology without impeding denaturation or subsequent hybridization (Binder *et al.* 1986; Fournier *et al.* 1991; Jiao *et al.*1992; Cennachi *et al.* 1993; Morey *et al.* 1993).

Fixation in osmium tetroxide is incompatible with embedding in hydrophilic resins and has generally been found to impede hybridization (Mandry *et al.* 1993). There has been one report of successful hybridization to osmicated araldite-embedded tissue following pre-treatment with potassium periodate and etching with dilute, saturated, alcoholic sodium hydroxide, though labelling was still only 10% of that obtained in Lowicryl-embedded material (Lin *et al.* 1993).

Grids

Standard copper grids are unsuitable for mounting thin sections for ISH processing since the copper ions react with the formamide present in the hybridization buffer to produce large, electron-dense aggregates on the grid bars (Gwaltney *et al.* 1993). Nickel or gold grids are therefore used; usually with a supporting membrane such as Formvar (Puvion-Dutielleul and Puvion, 1989; Morey *et al.* 1993), parlodion (Binder *et al.* 1986), or collodion (Dirks *et al.* 1993) which is ideally further stabilized by a thin layer of carbon. We found the latter step to be particularly important when using LR White resin in order to stop the formation of 'wrinkles' during hybridization processing (see EM Protocol 1).

Pre-treatment of sections (EM Protocol 2)

Proteolytic digestion

Although proteolytic digestion is routinely employed in *in situ* hybridization studies at the light microscope level, its usefulness at the electron microscope (EM) level is debatable. Several authors have reported that proteolytic digestion has adverse effects on ultrastructural morphology without producing a substantial improvement in signal intensity (Troxler *et al.* 1990; Escaig-Haye *et al.* 1992; Morey *et al.* 1993). However, studies of DNA viruses such as adenovirus and herpes simplex, which produce large amounts of DNA-binding protein, prove the exception to this rule (Puvion-Dutilleul and Puvion, 1991a,b). DNA-binding proteins can cause artefactual binding of DNA probes and/or impede probe access to the viral DNA target. In such circumstances, proteolytic digestion can increase the specific signal while reducing non-specific binding (Puvion-Dutilleul and Puvion, 1991a,b).

DNase/RNase digestion

Nuclease digestions can play an important role in controlling the specificity of the hybridization (by selectively eliminating DNA or RNA) and in confirming the identity of the signal (Puvion-Dutilleul and Puvion, 1990a,b; 1991a,b; Morey *et al.* 1993). It should be borne in mind, however, that nuclease digestion is often incomplete.

Denaturation

A variety of different methods of denaturing double-stranded DNA targets have been employed, including alkali, acid, and heat (with and without formamide) (Puvion-Dutilleul and Puvion, 1989; Mandry *et al.* 1993; Morey *et al.* 1993). Four-minute incubation in 0.5M NaOH appears to give the best results in both resin sections and ultrathin cryosections (Puvion-Dutilleul and Puvion, 1989; Mandry *et al.* 1993; Morey *et al.* 1993), although the optimal procedure is likely to vary with the fixation protocol employed.

Probes

Plasmid-derived, double-stranded DNA probes and single-stranded RNA probes (riboprobes) have both been employed for ultrastrucutral viral localization. Riboprobes permit strand discrimination of the target and have been reported to give greater sensitivity and reduced background (Troxler *et al.* 1990), although an obvious disadvantage is the necessity for meticulous avoidance of RNase contamination. There are relatively few reports of the use of oligonucleotide probes for viral detection at the ultrastructural level (Baccetti *et al.* 1994; Somasundaran *et al.* 1994), with probe cocktails being required to achieve sufficient sensitivity.

Most ultrastructural ISH studies have employed biotin-labelled probes; however, endogenous biotin is a common cause of false-positive signal at the light microscope level, and at least one report describes artefactual signal owing to endogenous biotin at the EM level (Puvion-Dutilleul and Puvion, 1991a). Digoxigenin is gaining in popularity as an alternative non-isotopic probe label at the light microscope level, and there are now a number of reports on the use of digoxigenin-labelled probes for viral genome localization at the ultrastructural level (Troxler *et al.* 1992; Cennachi *et al.* 1993; Lin *et al.* 1993; Morey *et al.* 1993, 1995; Egger *et al.* 1994). Digoxigenin does not occur endogenously in animal tissues, and comparative studies at the EM level indicate that digoxigenin-labelled probes are at least equal in sensitivity to biotin-labelled probes (Dirks *et al.* 1992; Egger *et al.* 1994).

Non-isotopic codetection of more than one target is possible by employing dual probe hybridization; this has been used to permit simultaneous detection of two portions of the poliovirus RNA genome using biotin- and digoxigenin-labelled probes and antibodies conjugated to gold colloids of different sizes for visualization (Troxler *et al.* 1992).

Hybridization

Ultrastructural hybridization protocols (see EM Protocol 3) generally employ a standard hybridization mixture containing 50% formamide and 10% dextran sulfate at a hybridization temperature of 37 °C. Dirks *et al.* (1992) found that the dextran sulfate did not have a beneficial effect on labelling, but did have an adverse effect on morphology; it was therefore omitted from their hybridization mix. Recommended hybridization times have varied from one (Puvion-Dutilleul *et al.* 1989; Mandry *et al.* 1993) to 18 hours (Escaig-Haye *et al.* 1992). Binder *et al.* (1986) found that the strength of labelling did not increase after 5 h, and there is a general perception that prolonged incubation in formamide-containing solutions may impair morphology. However, in a formal analysis of hybridization time vs. signal strength, Escaig-Haye *et al.* (1991) found that hybridization was maximal at 9 h, with most of the morphological deterioration occurring in the first hour. We found that hybridization times over 4 h were associated with absorption of water vapour by the hybridization mixture; therefore, hybridization time was routinely limited to 4 h.

Post-hybridization stringency washes in formamide are frequently employed at the light microscope level; however, at the ultrastructural level they have been shown to have an adverse effect on morphology and to produce various artefacts (Binder *et al.* 1986; Mandry *et al.* 1993). Resin sections fortunately do not appear to have the same propensity for non-specific probe binding as paraffin sections, and post-hybridization rinses in buffer with detergent (rather than formamide) appear to give adequate specificity.

Detection of probe

The commercial availability of antibodies conjugated to colloidal gold particles of defined size has been one of the major factors in the spread of ultrastructural ISH techniques. Although DAB substrate (with or without metallic enhancement) can be visualized at the EM level, it provides poor target resolution and cannot be quantified (Tsutsumi *et al.* 1991; Yun and Sherwood, 1992). The recent availability of 1 nm gold conjugates (which are visualized by silver amplification) may provide an alternative means of labelling in circumstances where penetration of reagents is difficult (i.e. in pre-embedding protocols), although silver amplification can result in particles of uneven size (Troxler *et al.* 1990; Egger *et al.* 1994).

The use of colloidal gold conjugates permits semi-quantitative analysis of signal, although the number of particles associated with any one target molecule will depend on the probe type, the number of steps in the detection protocol, and the size of the gold particles (higher labelling densities being found with particles of smaller size). Particles less than 10 nm in diameter are difficult to visualize when examining sections at low power, thus most workers have employed antibodies conjugated to 10 or 15 nm colloidal gold particles.

Numerous studies have found that two- or three-step immunodetection protocols (see EM Protocol 4) provide much greater sensivity than single-step detection; in particular, the use of direct avidin– or streptavidin–gold conjugates to detect biotin-labelled probes has been found to be unsuccessful by several groups (Troxler *et al.* 1990; Wenderoth and Eisenberg, 1991; Gwaltney *et al.* 1993). This has been suggested to be due to negative charge repulsion between target nucleic acids and colloidal gold particles (Wenderoth and Eisenberg, 1991), although successful direct detection of biotinylated probes has been achieved using an anti-biotin colloidal gold conjugate (Egger *et al.* 1994). Protein A–gold can be used instead of a secondary antibody, being capable of binding to the Fc portion of immunoglobulins of a variety of different species (Roth, 1982; Binder *et al.* 1986; Morey *et al.* 1993). The optical density of the gold conjugate should be checked before use; we found an optical density of 0.06 at 520 nm to be optimal.

Examination of sections (EM Protocol 5)
Tissue sections exposed to pre-embedding ISH are routinely osmicated after hybridization before standard embedding in plastic (Wolber *et al.* 1988, 1989). Since osmication of tissue is not possible prior to embedding in hydrophilic resins, sections require staining prior to examination after hybridization. Aqueous uranyl acetate is most frequently employed, sometimes with the addition of lead citrate, although Puvion-Dutilleul (1993) advises against the use of lead citrate on Lowicryl K4M sections, since the granularity of the resin is accentuated. Some authors advocate post-fixation in glutaraldehyde before counterstaining to minimize loss of gold signal (Troxler *et al.* 1990).

Interpretation of signal
The eventual strength of labelling is dependent on a wide variety of factors, and, as in any ISH experiment, rigorous control experiments are required in order to be able to interpret the results accurately. A list of appropriate controls is presented in Table 9.5. An estimate of the signal-to-noise ratio of a particular protocol can obviously be obtained by comparing particle counts over infected and non-infected cells (Jiao *et al.* 1992). The size of gold particle

Table 9.5 Controls

Negative controls	Positive controls
Use of heterologous, similarly labelled probe	Detection of previously localized, high copy
Omission of denaturation (if probing for DNA)	sequence
Sense-strand if using riboprobes	Known positive tissues
DNase/RNase digestions (NB. often incomplete)	Codetection of protein product
Omission of primary antibody	
Presence of known negative cells in section	
Known negative tissues	

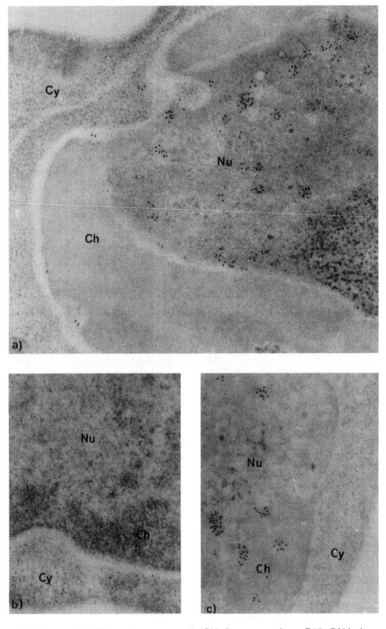

Fig. 9.1. (a) Post-embedding ultrastructural ISH for parvovirus B19 DNA in a fetal erythroid cell infected *in vitro*, embedded in LR White resin; digoxigenin-labelled DNA probe (pTY104; gift of Dr P. Tattersall), three-step immunodetection with 10 nm colloidal gold label. (b) Negative control probe, digoxigenin-labelled plasmid pBR322, 10 nm gold label. (c) Positive control probe, digoxigenin-labelled whole human DNA, 10 nm gold label; note labelling over marginated chromatin.

clusters appears to be an important factor in the differentiation of true hybridization signal from background; since a false-positive signal is usually a result of the immunodetection protocol rather than the hybridization *per se*, a false-positive signal is likely to be composed of single particles rather than clusters (Escaig-Haye *et al.* 1991).

Typical results on the localization of parovirus B19 DNA using a digoxigenin-labelled probe detected with a three-step immunodetection protocol (Morey *et al.* 1993) are shown in Fig. 9.1a. Results with the negative control probe (pBR322) and positive control probe (whole human DNA) are shown in Fig. 9.1b, respectively.

Combined ultrastructural *in situ* hybridization and immunocytochemistry

Non-isotopic ISH at the ultrastructural level is readily combined with immunocytochemical labelling of proteins, provided that the protein targets survive the embedding and hybridization processing, and provided the target nucleic acid does not require strong denaturation. Combination protocols have been used to co-localize HIV-I RNA plus core proteins p24 and p17 (Escaig-Haye *et al.* 1992), poliovirus RNA plus P2 and P3 proteins (Troxler *et al.* 1992), and parvovirus B19 DNA plus capsid and non-structural proteins (Morey *et al.* 1995). The antibody labelling is best performed after the hybridization procedure (the reverse order being usual at the light microscope level), either simultaneously with detection of the probe label (Escaig-Haye *et al.* 1992; Troxler *et al.* 1992) or as a sequential procedure (Morey *et al.* 1995). The gold colloids used to visualize each target should be sufficiently different in size that confusion is avoided. The three studies noted above all employed resin-embedded cells, although co-localization of non-viral mRNA and protein targets has also been achieved in whole-mount cells (Singer *et al.* 1989) and frozen sections (Dirks *et al.* 1992, 1993).

We found that the parvovirus B19 genome could be readily co-localized with the viral capsid and non-structural proteins (Morey *et al.* 1995), since the single-stranded B19 virion DNA did not require denaturation (which can adversely affect the integrity of proteins). Triple labelling of all three targets was a theoretical possibility, although practical difficulties in avoiding species cross-reactivity between secondary and tertiary antibodies used for detection of each different target produced less than optimal results. Typical results on the co-localization of B19 DNA and capsid protein are shown in Fig. 9.2.

Conclusions

Non-isotopic *in situ* hybridization at the ultrastructural level provides a rapid and highly specific means of examining aspects of intracellular viral nucleic acid metabolism. The various hybridization methods have different advan-

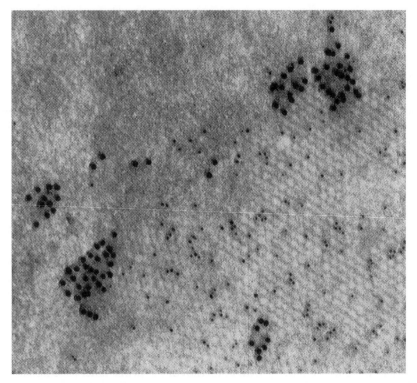

Fig. 9.2. Combined ultrastructural ISH/ICC for parvovirus B19 DNA (digoxigenin-labelled DNA probe, three-step detection with 10 nm gold label) and parvovirus capsid antigen (antibody R92F6; gift of Dr H. O'Neill, two-step detection with 5 nm gold label) over a paracrystalline array of viral particles.

tages and disadvantages, with sensitivity and morphological preservation being mutually opposed. The choice of protocol will therefore depend on the particular requirements of the question under investigation. The technique is highly specific rather than highly sensitive, and a target that cannot be detected at the light microscope level is unlikely to be successfully localized at the EM level. *In situ* hybridization is readily combined with immunocytochemical labelling of proteins (provided the antigenicity of the protein targets is retained during the hybridization processing) and the combination of these two techniques provides a powerful means of examining intracellular viral life cycles.

References

Baccetti, B., Benedetto, A., Burrini, A.G., Collodel, G., Ceccarini E., *et al.* (1994). HIV-1 particles in spermatazoa of patients with AIDS and their transfer into the oocyte. *J. Cell Biol.*, **127**, 903–14.

Combined in situ *hybridization and immunocytochemistry*

Balluz, I.M., Glasgow, G.M., Killen, H.M., Mabruk, M.J., Sheahan, B.J., and Atkins, G.J. (1993). Virulent and avirulent strains of Semliki Forest virus show similar cell tropism for the murine central nervous system but differ in the severity and rate of induction of cytolytic damage. *Neuropathol. Appl. Neurobiol.*, **19**, 233–9.

Besse, S. and Puvion-Dutilleul, F. (1994). Compartmentalization of cellular and viral DNAs in adenovirus type 5 infection as revealed by ultrastructural *in situ* hybridization. *Chromosome Res.*, **2**, 123–35.

Besse, S., Vigmeron, M., Pichard, E., and Puvion-Dutilleul, F. (1995). Synthesis and maturation of viral transcripts in herpes simplex virus type I infected HeLa cells: the role of interchromatin granules. *Gene Expr.*, **4**, 143–61.

Bienz, K., Egger, D., Pfister, T., and Troxler, M. (1992). Structural and functional characterization of the poliovirus replication complex. *J. Virol.*, **66**, 2740–7.

Binder, M., Tourmente, S., Roth, J., Renaud, M., and Gehring, W.J. (1986). *In situ* hybridization at the electron microscope level: localization of transcripts in ultrathin sections of Lowicryl K4M-embedded tissue using biotinylated probes and protein A–gold complexes. *J. Cell Biol.*, **102**, 1646–53.

Blum, H.E., Haase, A.T., and Vyas, G.N. (1984). Molecular pathogenesis of hepatitis B virus infection: simultaneous detection of viral DNA and antigens in paraffin-embedded liver sections. *Lancet*, **ii**, 771–5.

Brahic, M. and Haase, A.T. (1978). Detection of viral sequences of low reiteration frequency by *in situ* hybridization. *Proc. Natl. Acad. Sci. USA*, **75**, 6125–9.

Brahic, M., Haase, A.T. and Cash, E. (1984). Simultaneous *in situ* detection of viral RNA and antigens. *Proc. Natl. Acad. Sci. USA*, **81**, 5445–8.

Cenacchi, G., Musiani, M., Gentilomi, G., Righi, S., Zerbini, M., Chandler, J.G., Scala, C., Placa, M.L., and Martinelli, G.N. (1993). *In situ* hybridization at the ultrastructural level: localization of cytomegalovirus DNA using digoxigenin labelled probes. *J. Submicrosc. Cytol. Pathol.*, **25**, 341–5.

Croissant, O., Dauguet, C., Jeanteur, P., and Orth, G. (1972). Application de la technique d'hybridation moleculaire in situ a la mise en evidence au microscope electronique de la replication vegetative de l'ADN viral dans les papillomes provoques par le virus de Shope chez lapin cottontail. *C. R. Acad. Sci.*, **274**, 614–18.

Dirks, R.W., van Dorp, A.G., van Minnen, J., Fransen, J.A., van der Ploeg, M., and Raap, A. K. (1992). Electron microscopic detection of RNA sequences by non-radioactive *in situ* hybridization in the mollusk *Lymnaea stagnalis*. *J. Histochem. Cytochem.*, **40**, 1647–57.

Dirks, R.W., van Dorp, A.G., van Minnen, J., Fransen, J.A., van der Ploeg, M., and Raap, A. K. (1993). Ultrastructural evidence for the axonal localization of caudodorsal cell hormone mRNA in the central nervous system of the mollusc *Lymnaea stagnalis*. *Microsc. Res. Tech.*, **25**, 12–18.

Egger, D., Troxler, M., and Bienz, K. (1994). Light and electron microscopic *in situ* hybridization; non-radioactive labelling and detection, double hybridization and combined hybridization-immunohistochemistry. *J. Histochem. Cytochem.*, **42**, 815–22.

Escaig-Haye, F., Grigoriev, V., Peranzi, G., Lestienne, P., and Fournier, J.G. (1991). Analysis of human mitochondrial transcripts using electron microscopic *in situ* hybridization. *J. Cell Sci.*, **100**, 851–62.

Escaig-Haye, F., Grigoriev, V., Sharova, I., Rudneva, V., Buckrinskaya, A., and Fournier, J.G. (1992). Ultrastructural localization of HIV-1 RNA and core proteins.

Simultaneous visualization using double immunogold labelling after *in situ* hybridization and immunocytochemistry. *J. Submicrosc. Cytol. Pathol.*, **24**, 437–43.

Fleming, K.A., Evans, M., Riley, K.C., Franklin, D., Lovell-Badge, R.H., and Morey, A.L. (1992). Optimisation of non-isotopic *in situ* hybridization on formalin-fixed paraffin-embedded material using digoxigenin labelled probes and transgenic tissues. *J. Pathol.*, **161**, 9–17.

Fournier, J.G., Escaig-Haye, F., and Grigoriev, V. (1991). Ultrastructural detection of cellular and viral RNA with biotinylated DNA probes. *Bull. Assoc. Anat.*, **75**, 13–15.

Gendelman, H.E., Moench, T.R., Naragan, O., Griffin, D.E., and Clemants, J.E. (1985). A double labelling technique for performing immunocytochemistry and *in situ* hybridisation in virus infected cell cultures and tissues. *J. Virol. Meth.*, **11**, 93.

Geuskens, M. and May, E. (1974). Ultrastructural localization of SV40 viral DNA in cells during lytic infection, by *in situ* molecular hybridization. *Exp. Cell Res.*, **87**, 175.

Gosztonyi, G., Artigas, J., Lamperth, L., and Webster, H.D. (1994). Human immunodeficiency virus (HIV) distribution in HIV encephalitis: study of 19 cases with combined use of *in situ* hybridization and immunocytochemistry. *J. Neuropathol. Exp. Neurol.*, **53**, 521–34.

Graham, A.K., Herrington, C.S., and McGee, J.O'D. (1991). Simultaneous *in situ* genotyping and phenotyping of human papillomavirus cervical lesions: comparative sensitivity and specificity. *J. Clin. Pathol.*, **44**, 96–101.

Guinee, D., Jr, Jaffe, E., Kingma, D., Fishback, N., Wallberg, K., Krishnan, J., Frizzera, G., Travis, W., and Koss, M. (1994). Pulmonary lymphomatoid granulomatosis. Evidence for a proliferation of Epstein–Barr virus infected B-lymphocytes with a prominent T-cell component and vasculitis. *Am. J. Surg. Pathol.*, **18**, 753–64.

Gwaltney, S.M., Willard, L.H., and Oberst, R.D. (1993). *In situ* hybridization of *Eperythrozoon suis* visualized by electron microscopy. *Vet. Microbiol.*, **36**, 99–112.

Hagari, Y., Shibata, M., Mihara, M., Shimao, S., and Kurimura, T. (1993). Detection of human papillomavirus type 2a DNA in verrucae vulgares by electron microscopic *in situ* hybridization. *Arch. Dermatol. Res.*, **285**, 255–260.

Ironside, J.W., Lewis, F.A., Blythe, D., and Wakefield, E.A. (1989). The identification of cells containing JC papovavirus DNA in progressive multifocal leukoencephalopathy by combined *in situ* hybridisation and immunocytochemistry. *J. Pathol.*, **157**, 291–7.

Jiao, R., Yu, W., Ding, M., and Zhai, Z. (1992). Localization of adenovirus DNA by *in situ* hybridization electron microscopy. *Microsc. Res. Tech.*, **21**, 23–31.

Jiwa, N.M., Kanavoaros, P., de Bruin, P.C., van der Valk, P., Horstman, A., Vos, W., Mullink, H., Walboomers, J.M., and Meijer, C.J. (1993). Presence of Epstein–Barr virus harbouring small and intermediate-sized cells in Hodgkin's disease. Is there a relationship with Reed–Stern berg cells? *J. Pathol.*, **170**, 129–36.

Lau, J.Y.N., Naoumov, N.V., Alexander, G.J.M., and Williams, R. (1991). Rapid detection of hepatitis B virus DNA in liver tissue by *in situ* hybridisation and its combination with immunohistochemistry for simultaneous detection of HBV antigens. *J. Clin. Pathol.*, **44**, 905–8.

Lin, N.S., Chen, C.C., and Hsu, Y.H. (1993). Post-embedding *in situ* hybridization for localization of viral nucleic acid in ultra-thin sections. *J. Histochem. Cytochem.*, **41**, 1513–19.

Mandry, P., Murray, B.A., Rieke, L., Becke, H., and Hofler, H. (1993). Postembedding ultrastructural *in situ* hybridization on ultrathin cryosections and LR white resin sections. *Ultrastruct. Pathol.*, **17**, 185–94.

McQuaid, S., Allen, I.V., McMahon, J., and Kirk, J. (1994). Association of measles virus with neurofibrillary tangles in subacute sclerosing panencephalitis: a combined *in situ* hybridization and immunocytochemical investigation. *Neuropath. Appl. Neurobiol.*, **20**, 103–10.

Morey, A.L. and Fleming, K.A. (1992). Immunophenotyping of fetal haematopoietic cells permissive for human parvovirus (B19) replication *in vitro. Br. J. Haematol.*, **82**, 302–9.

Morey, A.L., Porter, H.J., Keeling, J.W., and Fleming, K.A. (1992). Non-isotopic *in situ* hybridisation and immunophenotyping of infected cells in the investigation of human fetal parvovirus infection. *J. Clin. Pathol.*, **45**, 673–8.

Morey, A.L., Ferguson, D.J., Leslie, K.O., Taatjes, D.J., and Fleming, K.A. (1993). Intracellular localization of parvovirus B19 nucleic acid at the ultrastructural level by *in situ* hybridization with digoxigenin-labelled probes. *Histochem. J.*, **25**, 421–9.

Morey, A.L., Fergson, D.J.P., and Fleming, K.A. (1995). Combined immunocyto-chemistry and non-isotopic *in situ* hybridization for the ultrastructural investigation of human parvovirus B19 infection. *Histochem. J.*, **27**, 46–53.

Mullink, H., Walboomers, J.M.M., Tadema, T.M., Jansen, D.J., and Meijer, C.J. (1989). Combined immuno- and non-radioactive hybridocytochemistry on cells and tissue sections: influence of fixation, enzyme pre-treatment and choice of chromogen on detection of antigen and DNA sequences. *J. Histochem. Cytochem.*, **37**, 603–9.

Multhaupt, H.A., Rafferty, P.A., and Warhol, M.J. (1992). Ultrastructural localization of human papilloma virus by nonradioactive *in situ* hybridization on tissue of human cervical intraepithelial neoplasia. *Lab. Invest.*, **67**, 512–18.

Myerson, D., Hachman, R.C., Nelson, J.A., Ward, D.C., and McDougal, J.K. (1984). Widespread presence of histologically occult cytomegalovirus. *Hum. Pathol.*, **15**, 430–9.

Porter, H.J., Heryet, A., Quantrill, A.M., and Fleming, K.A. (1990). Combined non-isotopic *in situ* hybridisation and immunohistochemistry on routine paraffin wax embedded tissue: identification of cell type infected by human parvovirus and demonstration of cytomegalovirus DNA and antigen in viral infection. *J. Clin. Pathol.*, **43**, 129–32.

Puvion-Dutilleul, F. (1993). Procedures of *in situ* nucleic acid hybridization to detect viral DNA and RNA in cells by electron microscopy. In: *Hybridization techniques for electron microscopy*, (ed. G. Morel), pp. 269–300. CRC Press, Boca Raton.

Puvion-Dutilleul, F. and Pichard, E. (1992). Segregation of viral double-stranded and single-stranded DNA molecules in nuclei of adenovirus infected cells as revealed by electron microscope *in situ* hybridization. *Biol. Cell*, **76**, 139–50.

Puvion-Dutilleul, F. and Pichard, E. (1993). Superiority of *in situ* hybridization over immunolabelling for detecting DNA on Lowicryl sections: a study on adenovirus-infected cells. *J. Histochem. Cytochem.*, **41**, 1537–46.

Puvion-Dutilleul, F. and Puvion, E. (1989). Ultrastructural localization of viral DNA in thin sections of herpes simplex virus type 1 infected cells by *in situ* hybridization. *Eur. J. Cell Biol.*, **49**, 99–109.

Puvion-Dutilleul, F. and Puvion, E. (1990a). Replicating single-stranded adenovirus type 5 DNA molecules accumulate within well-delimited intranuclear areas of lytically infected HeLa cells. *Eur. J. Cell Biol.*, **52**, 379–88.

Puvion-Dutilleul, F. and Puvion, E. (1990b). Analysis by *in situ* hybridization and autoradiography of sites of replication and storage of single- and double-stranded adenovirus type 5 DNA in lytically infected HeLa cells. *J. Struct. Biol.*, **103**, 280–9.

In situ *Hybridization*

Puvion-Dutilleul, F. and Puvion, E. (1991a). Ultrastructural localization of defined sequences of viral RNA and DNA by *in situ* hybridization of biotinylated DNA probes on sections of herpes simplex virus type 1 infected cells. *J. Electron Microsc. Tech.*, **18**, 336–53.

Puvion-Dutilleul, F. and Puvion, E. (1991b). Sites of transcription of adenovirus type 5 genomes in relation to early viral DNA replication in infected HeLa cells. A high resolution *in situ* hybridization and autoradiographical study. *Biol. Cell*, **71**, 135–47.

Puvion-Dutilleul, F., Pichard, E., Laithier, M., and Puvion, E. (1989). Cytochemical study of the localization and organization of parental herpes simplex virus type I DNA during initial infection of the cell. *Eur. J. Cell Biol.*, **50**, 187–200.

Puvion-Dutilleul, F., Roussev, R., and Puvion E. (1992). Distribution of viral RNA molecules during the adenovirus type 5 infectious cycle in HeLa cells. *J. Struct. Biol.*, **108**, 209–20.

Roberts, W.H., Sneddon, J.M., Waldman, J., and Stephens, R.E. (1989). Cytomegalovirus infection of gastrointestinal endothelium demonstrated by simultaneous nucleic acid hybridization and immunohistochemistry. *Arch. Pathol. Lab. Med.*, **113**, 461–84.

Roth, J. (1982). The protein A-gold (pAg) technique—a qualitative and quantitative approach for antigen localization on thin sections. In: *Techniques in immunocytochemistry*, Vol. 1, (ed. G.R. Bullock and P. Petrusz), pp. 108–30. Academic Press, London.

Singer, R.H., Langevin, G.L., and Lawrence, J.B. (1989). Ultrastructural visualization of cytoskeletal mRNAs and their associated proteins using double-label *in situ* hybridization. *J. Cell Biol.*, **108**, 2343–53.

Somasundaran, M., Zapp, M.L., Beattie, L.K., Pang, L., Byron, K.S., Bassell, G.J., Sullivan, J.L., and Singer, R.H. (1994). Localization of HIV RNA in mitochondria of infected cells: potential role in cytopathogenicity. *J. Cell Biol.*, **126**, 1353–60.

Troxler, M., Pasamontes, L., Egger, D., and Bienz, K. (1990). *In situ* hybridization for light and electron microscopy: a comparison of methods for the localization of viral RNA using biotinylated DNA and RNA probes. *J. Virol. Meth*, **30**, 1–14.

Troxler, M., Egger, D., Pfister, T., and Bienz, K. (1992). Intracellular localization of poliovirus RNA by *in situ* hybridization at the ultrastructural level using single-stranded riboprobes. *Virology*, **191**, 687–97.

Tsutsumi, Y., Kawai, K., Hori, S., and Osamura, R.Y. (1991). Ultrastructural visualization of human papillomavirus DNA in verrucopus and precancerous squamous lesions. *Acta Pathol. Jpn*, **41**, 757–62.

van der Loos, C.M., Vokers, H.H., Rook, R., van den Berg, F.M., and Houthoff, H.J. (1989). Simultaneous application of *in situ* DNA hybridisation and immunohistochemistry on one tissue section. *Histochem. J.*, **21**, 279–84.

Wenderoth, M.P. and Eisenberg, B.R. (1991). Ultrastructural distribution of myosin heavy chain mRNA in cardiac tissue: a comparison of frozen and LR White embedment. *J. Histochem. Cytochem.*, **39**, 1025–33.

Wolber, R.A., Beals, T.F., Lloyd, R.V., and Maassab, H.F. (1988). Ultrastructural localization of viral nucleic acid by *in situ* hybridization. *Lab. Invest.*, **59**, 144–51.

Wolver, R.A., Beals, T.F., and Maassab, H.F. (1989). Ultrastructural localization of herpes simplex virus RNA by *in situ* hybridization. *J. Histochem. Cytochem.*, **37**, 97–104.

Yoshioka, M., Shapsak, P., Sun, N.C., Nelson, S.J., Svenningsson, A., Tate, L.G., Pardo, V., and Resnick, L. (1992). Simultaneous detection of ferritin and HIV-1 in reactive microglia. *Acta Neuropathol.*, **84**, 297–306.
Yun, K. and Sherwood, M.J. (1992). *In situ* hybridization at light and electron misroscopic levels: identification of human papillomavirus nucleic acids. *Pathology*, **24**, 91–8.

Appendix 9.1

Protocol for combined non-isotopic in situ hybridization/immunocytochemistry at the LM level

All manipulations should be performed in nuclease-free containers.

Immunocytochemistry (modified APPAP protocol)

1. Cut 5 μm sections on to silane treated slides, air dry (no more than overnight), then back at 80 °C for 30–120 min.

2. Dewax sections in xylene immediately before use and take to distilled autoclaved water via graded alcohols.

3. Perform protease digestion if required [e.g. 0.05 mg/ml protease VIII (Sigma) in phosphate buffer saline, 20 min at room temperature]; pre-incubation of protease solution at 37 °C for 30 minutes is advised prior to application to sections in order to autodigest nucleases.

4. Wash sections in Tris buffer saline (TBS; 150 mM NaCl, 50 mM Tris; pH 7.2) at room temperature, 3 × 3 min.

5. Apply primary antibody (e.g. mouse monoclonal) for 60 min at room temperature, diluted appropriately in TBS with 1% bovine serum albumin (BSA).

6. Wash sections in TBS, 3 × 3 min.

7. Apply secondary bridging antibody (e.g. rabbit anti-mouse immuno-globulins), diluted as appropriate, for 30 min at room temperature.

8. Wash slides in TBS, 3 × 3 min.

9. Apply alkaline phosphatase anti-alkaline phosphatase conjugate (APAAP), diluted as appropriate for 30 min at room temperature.

10. Wash slides in TBS, 3 × 3 min.

11. Incubate slides in substrate (e.g. Fast Red/Napthol-AS-MX phosphate) and monitor by microscopy (about 30 min room temperature).

12. Rinse off substrate in distilled autoclaved water and stored in autoclaved ice-cold TBS for up to 24 h (do not allow to dry).

In situ *Hybridization*

In situ hybridization

1. Remove sections from TBS and rinse well in autoclaved water.

2. Perform protease digestion for *in situ* hybridization (if no protease digestion was performed in immunocytochemistry section) then rinse well in autoclaved water.

3. Denature target DNA by immersing sections in autoclaved water at 95°C for 10 min, cool rapidly in ice-cold autoclaved water, then allow to air dry.

4. Dissolve digoxigenin-labelled DNA probes (see Fleming *et al.* 1992) at a final concentration of 1 μg/ml in hybridization mixture consisting of 10% dextran sulfate, 50% deionized formamide, 250 μg/ml sheared herring sperm DNA, 0.01% polyvinylpyrrolidine, 0.1% sodium dodecyl sulfate in 2 × SET buffer (300 mM NaCl, 60 mM Tris, 4 mM EDTA; pH 7.0). Denature probes at 95°C for 15 min, snap freeze on dry ice or liquid nitrogen, then keep at 0°C until use.

5. Apply probes (including appropriate controls) to sections under 18 mm^2 coverslips (7.5 μl per section) and seal the edges with silicone grease. Hybridize for 2 h at 37°C in a moist chamber.

6. Remove coverslips in modified Tris-buffered saline (MTBS: 15 mM Tris, 150 mM NaCl; pH 7.6) with 0.5% Triton-X100 then wash 3 × 5 min in the same solution at 37°C.

7. Perform stringency washes in 0.5 × MTBS for 3 × 3 minutes at 65°C and remove any remaining silicone grease.

8. Block non-specific protein binding with 15% skimmed milk powder in AP7.5 buffer (0.1 M Tris, 0.1 M NaCl, 2 mM MgCl$_2$; pH 7.5) with 0.5% Triton for 15 min at 37°C.

9. After rinsing briefly in AP7.5 buffer, apply sheep polyclonal anti-digoxigenin conjugated with alkaline phosphatase (Boehringer Mannheim) diluted 1:750 in 2% bovine serum albumin in AP7.5/0.5% Triton for 30 min at 37°C.

10. Remove unbound conjugate by 3 × 5 min rinses in AP7.5/0.5% Triton, then 3 × 3 min rinses in AP9.0 buffer (0.1 M Tris, 0.1 M NaCl, 0.1 M MgCl$_2$; pH 9.0).

11. Immerse sections in NBT/BCIP substrate in a light-shielded container. After development of signal (monitor by microscopy), rinse slides in dH$_2$O and mount in Kaiser's glycerol jelly.

EM Protocol 1.   Preparation of resin sections of cells

1. Pellet cell suspension (approx. 2.5×10^6 cells per tube; 5 min at 250 *g*).

2. Fix cell pellets for 30 min in freshly prepared 2% paraformaldehyde/0.1% glutaraldehyde in 0.1 M phosphate buffer (pH 7.2) at 37°C, cooling gradually to room temperature.

3. Pellet cells (5 min at 250*g*) then wash thoroughly in phosphate buffer before repelleting.

4. Dehydrate cell pellets in increasing concentrations of chilled ethanol over a period of 4 h in the freezer and embed in LR White resin. The steps involved are:

50% ethanol	15 min	(−20°C)
70% ethanol	15 min	(−20°C)
90% ethanol	15 min	(−20°C)
100% ethanol	15 min	(−20°C)
100% ethanol/LR White (1:1)	3 hours	(−20°C)
100% LR White	overnight	(−20°C)
100% LR White	2 hours	(room temp).

5. Transfer pellets to gelatin capsules filled with fresh LR White resin and polymerise at 60°C for 18 h.

6. Cut thin sections on to carbon/Formvar-coated nickel grids (200 mesh).

7. Store at room temperature until required.

EM Protocol 2.   Pre-treatment of resin sections

Thin sections are processed by floating the grids, face down, on drops of the appropriate solutions placed on fresh Parafilm sheets. All solutions should be sterile and millipore filtered (0.2 μm pore size) in order to remove particulate debris.

1. Perform optional proteolytic digestion [protease VIII (Sigma) at 0.05 mg/ml in phosphate buffered saline (12 mM $Na_2HPO_4.2H_2O$, 40 mM KH_2PO_4, 150 mM NaCl; pH 7.2] for 20 min at room temperature.

2. Rinse 5×2 min in distilled autoclaved water (dH_2O).

3. Perform optional nuclease digestion [DNase and/or RNase A (Boehringer Mannheim) diluted 1 mg/ml in DNase buffer (50 mM Tris, 10 mM $MgCl_2$; pH 7.8) for 20 min at room temperature].

4. Rinse 5×2 min in dH_2O.

5. Perform optional denaturation (for double-stranded DNA target) in 0.5 M NaOH at room temperature for 5 min.

6. Rinse 5 × 2 min with dH$_2$O and air dry.

EM Protocol 3. Preparation and hybridization of digoxigenin-labelled probes

1. Nick translate double-stranded DNA probes with digoxigenin-11-dUTP (Boehringer Mannheim) to a mean fragment length of approximately 200 bases (see Fleming *et al.* 1992).

2. Add probes at a final concentration of 1 μg/ml to hybridization mix consisting of 10% dextran sulfate, 50% deionized formamide, 250 μg/ml sheared herring sperm DNA, 0.01% polyvinylpyrrolidine, 0.1% sodium dodecyl sulfate in 2 × SET buffer (300 mM NaCl, 4 mM EDTA, 50 mM Tris; pH 7.4).

3. Denature probe mixtures in eppendorf tubes suspended in hot water at 95 °C for 15 min then snap freeze and store on ice until use.

4. Hybridize thin sections by floating grids upside down on 20 μl drops of denatured probe mixture on a Parafilm sheet in a sealed, moist chamber at 37 °C for 4 h.

5. Perform post-hybridization washes (5 × 2 min at 37 °C) on drops of TBS (50 mM Tris, 150 mM NaCl; pH 7.2) containing 0.5% Triton.

6. Perform optional stringency washes (5 × 2 min at 42 °C) on drops of 0.5 × TBS containing 0.5% Triton.

EM Protocol 4. Three-step immunodetection of digoxigenin-labelled probes

Care should be taken to avoid drying of sections between steps.

1. Block non-specific protein binding with 1% bovine serum albumin (BSA) in TBS with 0.5% Triton (TBS/Triton/BSA) for 15 min at 37 °C.

2. Incubate in sheep polyclonal anti-digoxigenin antibody (Boehringer Mannheim) diluted to 2 μg/ml in TBS/Triton/BSA for 1 h at 37 °C.

3. Rinse 5 × 2 min rinses on drops of TBS.

4. Incubate in polyclonal rabbit anti-sheep antibody diluted to 25 μg/ml in TBS/Triton/BSA for 30 min at 37 °C.

5. Rinse 5 × 2 min rinses on drops of TBS.

6. Incubate in goat anti-rabbit antibody conjugated to 10 nm colloidal gold particles (Biocell: optical density of 3.0 at 520 nm) diluted 1:50 in TBS/ Triton/BSA.

7. Rinse 5 × 2 min rinses on drops of dH_2O.

8. Air dry.

EM Protocol 5.   Examination of sections

1. Counterstain sections with filtered 2% aqueous uranyl acetate (6 min).

2. Rinse 5 × 2 min rinses on drops of dH_2O.

3. Air dry completely prior to examination in electron microscope.

EM Protocol 6.   Immunocytochemical detection of viral proteins

This protocol may follow on directly from protocol 4, without allowing the grids to dry.

1. Block non-specific binding with 1% BSA in TBS with 0.5% Triton for 15 min at room temperature.

2. Incubate on drops of primary antibody (e.g. mouse monoclonal) diluted appropriately in TBS/1%BSA for 1 h at room temperature.

3. Rinse 5 × 2 min on drops of TBS.

4. Incubate on drops of secondary antibody conjugated to 5 nm gold conjugate [e.g. goat anti-mouse antibody (Biocell) diluted 1:25 in TBS/1%BSA] for 30 min at room temperature.

5. Rinse 5 × 2 min on drops of dH_2O.

6. Counterstain as above (Protocol 5).

10

Supersensitive *in situ* DNA and RNA localization

GERHARD W. HACKER, INGEBORG ZEHBE, and
RAYMOND TUBBS

Introduction

In situ detection of specific nucleic acid sequences is possible with a variety of *in situ* hybridization (ISH) methods, most of which are discussed in this book. Non-isotopic probes possess great advantages over radioactivity labelled probes; not only does the use of non-isotopic reporter molecules, such as biotin, digoxigenin, or fluorescent labels, make it possible to avoid hazardous radiation and to shorten the turnover period, but they also give an improved resolution and are more economic than radioisotopes. For this reason, biotin- or digoxigenin-labelled probes are frequently used for various purposes: in daily research and histopathological diagnosis to detect viral nucleic acids in infected cells, to investigate biosynthesis of peptides or proteins, to detect cancer genes, and to study genetic diseases (for reviews see this book and, for example, Giaid *et al.* 1989; Chan and McGee 1990; Polak and McGee 1990; Höfler 1990; Herrington and McGee 1992; Luke *et al.* 1997).

The drawback of conventional ISH is its detection limit of about 20 viral copies per cell (Zehbe *et al.* 1992a, 1993b). Latent viral infections or early pathological changes often involve fewer copies of nucleotide sequences than those detectable by conventional ISH alone. Using the *in vitro* polymerase chain reaction (PCR), minute quantities of DNA sequences can be amplified to millions of identical copies for analysis but cannot be correlated with morphology (Bagasra 1990; Haase *et al.* 1990; Nuovo 1991, 1992; Nuovo *et al.* 1991; Bagasra *et al.* 1992, 1994, 1995a,b,c, 1996; Komminoth *et al.* 1992; Komminoth and Long 1993; Long *et al.* 1993; Gu 1994; Hacker and Danscher 1994; Hacker *et al.* 1994, 1995, 1996a,b,c; Sällström *et al.* 1994; Martinez *et al.* 1997). A combination of this method with histochemical techniques, designated *in situ* PCR (IS-PCR), as was shown on SiHa cells, enables the detection of single copies of viral HPV DNA (Zehbe *et al.* 1992b, 1993a, 1994b,c, 1995), but shows a relatively high possibility of false-negative or even false-positive reactions (Komminoth *et al.* 1992; Komminoth and Long 1993; Long *et al.*

1993; Sällström *et al.* 1994; Hacker *et al.* 1996a,b, 1997; Zehbe *et al.* 1997). In most laboratories, reproducibility and specificity are low, and therefore, at this stage, we cannot recommend this method as a routine diagnostic procedure. Another technique relying on amplified DNA or RNA, called the *in situ* 3SR technique, was described by our group for the first time (Zehbe *et al.* 1994a,b). So far, only one other group has used a similar protocol (Höfler *et al.* 1995), but this technique is also quite complicated and expensive.

The search for alternative procedures that would be easier to use, more reliable, and less expensive was therefore needed. A series of new applications of molecular biology now allow the supersensitive detection of nucleic acid sequences *in situ* and provide fascinating new insights into infection and virus processing in the host cell. Potential uses include the detection of foreign genes (infections, introduced genes), altered genes (genetic disease), or gene expression (mRNA). Detection of genetic alterations is currently gaining in importance in an exponential manner, as discoveries of tumour-associated gene sequences grow rapidly. These recently described approaches can be performed routinely in laboratories, without the need for expensive equipment. They rely on amplification of the label, rather than on nucleid acid amplification. One of these approaches is streptavidin–Nanogold™–silver ISH, an easy to perform assay detecting low copy numbers of nucleic acid sequences in paraffin sections and cytology (Hacker *et al.* 1996a,b, 1997). This technique gives an intense black signal and often shows a higher number of positive cells than are detected by standard ISH (alkaline phosphatase and peroxidase) applied on parallel sections. In combination with labelled tyramides deposited on peroxidase molecules [TSA™, also known as CARD (catalysed reporter deposition)] (Bobrow *et al.* 1989, 1991; Kerstens *et al.* 1995; Zehbe *et al.* 1997) this method can achieve single gene copy sensitivity in detection DNA viruses and also gives the highest sensitivity for RNA ISH (Hacker *et al.* 1997; Zehbe *et al.* 1997; Tubbs *et al.* 1997a,b; Tbakhi *et al.* 1988; Totos *et al.* submitted). It maybe foreseen that such supersensitive ISH techniques can potentially replace IS-PCR and related methodologies, because they are, at this stage, more reliable, less cost-intensive, and easier to perform.

The sensitivity and outcome of ISH, IS-PCR, and related techniques depends, to a high degree, on the quality of the detection system applied. Our group has specialized in the use of silver-amplified gold labelling systems, earlier using colloidal gold adsorbed to macromolecules (Faulk and Taylor 1971), and most recently with the newly described *Nanogold™*, a gold cluster surrounded by organic molecules covalently bound to streptavidin (Hainfeld 1987, 1990; Troxler *et al.* 1990; Hainfeld and Furuja 1992;). These neutrally charged, tiny, gold particles, of only 1.4 nm in diameter, can easily penetrate into cellular structures and are subsequently amplified in size by a silver technique called autometallography (AMG), introduced by Danscher (Danscher 1981a,b, 1984), who was also the first person to demonstrate colloidal gold in tissue sections with AMG (Danscher and Norgaard 1983). The AMG set-up had earlier, misleadingly, been called 'physical development' or 'silver enhancement', and was applied by Danscher to detect catalytic metals and in enzyme histochemistry (Danscher 1981a,b, 1984; Danscher and Norgaard 1983; Danscher *et al.* 1993, 1995), while Holgate and colleagues used it for immunocytochemistry (immunogold–silver staining, IGSS) (Holgate *et al.* 1983). IGSS is highly sensitive and efficient, simple to perform, and gives a delicate black staining of the structures demonstrated (e.g. Holgate *et al.* 1983; Springall *et al.* 1984; Hacker *et al.* 1988, 1995, 1996c; Hacker and Danscher 1994). Using AMG, gold particles increase in size through silver precipitation and, if sufficiently adjacent to each other, they may conglomerate, resulting in a greyish to black precipitate on relevant sites visible by both light and electron microscopy (for reviews see Danscher *et al.* 1993, 1995; Hacker and Danscher 1994b; Hacker *et al.* 1995, 1996c). Silver acetate AMG (Hacker *et al* 1988) is an easy to perform, efficient, and economic AMG developer which is less sensitive to light than silver lactate, nitrate, or bromide AMG, thus allowing the monitoring of the amplification process under light microscopical control (Hacker *et al.* 1995). ISH had been successfully combined with IGSS detection for more than a decade already (e.g. Varndell *et al.* 1984; Jackson *et al.* 1990; Hacker *et al.* 1993, 1994, 1995, 1996a,b,c, 1997; Hacker and Danscher 1994).

In the following text, the advantages and disadvantages of the IS-PCR techniques presently used are discussed. Following this, streptavidin–Nanogold–silver ISH with and without CARD amplification is presented and the appendix gives suggested step-by-step laboratory protocols.

In situ polymerase chain reaction (IS-PCR)

IS-PCR was first employed by Haase *et al.* 1990 and has undergone significant evolution since. The possibility of leaking amplicons during the amplification procedure was soon realized, and, in order to prevent this, different approaches were suggested. Haase *et al.* (1990) used multiple, overlapping primers which, so they argued, would result in long amplicons of approximately 900–1200 bp. Reasoning in the same way, Chiu *et al.* (1992) developed a system employing complementary primer tails. Nuovo (1991) and Nuovo *et al.* (1991) reported successful experiments at first using multiple primer pairs and later only one primer pair, and a 'hot start' PCR. Bagasra (1990) and Bagasra *et al.* (1992, 1994) approached the problem by using an additional fixation step prior to protease treatment and heating the samples to 95 °C after the actual PCR process. Finally, an assay was developed by Long *et al.* (1993) where diffusion artefacts are supposedly reduced by incorporating biotinylated nucleotides during polymerization to generate bulkier and therefore less diffusible amplicons. Single copies or low quantities of DNA or RNA can be amplified inside cytological or histological preparations. The aim has been to demon-strate specific nucleic acid sequences together with cell morphology.

From the first descriptions of IS-PCR by Bagasra (1990) and by Haase *et al.* (1990), a number of teams have reported their techniques over the years, and new insights into the distribution of low copy number nucleotide sequences have opened new possibilities for basic research and clinical diagnosis (e.g. Nuovo, 1991, 1992, 1996a,b; Nuovo *et al.* 1991; Bagasra *et al.* 1992, 1994, 1995a,b,c, 1996; Komminoth *et al.* 1992; Zehbe *et al.* 1992b, 1993a, 1994a,b,c, 1995; Komminoth and Long 1993; Long *et al.* 1993; Gu 1994; Hacker *et al.* 1994, 1995, 1996b; Sällström *et al.* 1994; Martinez *et al.* 1997). IS-PCR does not require a tedious DNA extraction, there is less risk for cross-sample con-tamination, and it appeared to be an uncompromised way to assess the morphology of positive and negative structures. Driven by numerous enthusiastic reports, we applied IS-PCR (Zehbe *et al.* 1992b) using human papillomavirus (HPV) as a model system. To optimize the technology and to act as a check of sensitivity, we used SiHa cell cultures derived from human cervical carcinoma, with only one to two copies of HPV type 16 per cell, one copy integrated into the host genome, and one copy as plasmid (Friedl *et al.* 1970; Zehbe *et al.* 1992b, 1993a, 1994a,b,c, 1995; Hacker *et al.* 1994, 1995, 1996b). In addition to numerous other modifications, we applied immunogold–silver staining (IGSS) for the first time, using colloidal gold (Zehbe *et al.* 1992b), and later the far superior Nanogold, as the label (Hacker *et al.* 1996a,b). Detection of the reporter molecules digoxigenin or biotin by IGSS showed a more distinct and high contrasting labelling (Fig. 10.1), and no hazardous reagent like DAB or radioactivity had to be used.

Earlier on, and also a number of recent papers on IS-PCR described the direct method (e.g. Zehbe *et al.* 1992b; Gu 1994; Martinez *et al.* 1997), in which a reporter molecule is incorporated directly into the newly synthesized DNA. Direct IS-PCR is easy to use, and, at that time, appeared to be a very specific set-up. However, it is common knowledge today that indirect tech-niques (Bagasra *et al.* 1992, 1994, 1995a,b,c, 1996; Nuovo 1992; Komminoth *et al.* 1992; Komminoth and Long 1993; Long *et al.* 1993; Zehbe *et al.* 1993a, 1994a,b,c, 1995; Gu 1994; Hacker *et al.* 1994, 1995, 1996b; Sällström *et al.* 1994) should be preferred, to avoid the false-positive reactions quite often associ-ated with direct IS-PCR. Mispriming of the DNA breakdown products contained in several types of cells, e.g. apoptotic cells, can cause non-specific incorporation of reporter molecules (Sällström *et al.* 1994), and indirect methods overcome these problems by carrying out a specific ISH following the PCR amplification (Nuovo 1991; Zehbe *et al.* 1993a).

Years of hands-on experience with IS-PCR, however, have shown that there are additional limitations with nearly all the IS-PCR systems available at present. A new and probably severe problem that was recognized recently is that of diffusion artefacts. Analyses of the liquid phase overlaying the preparations during the actual PCR process by electrophoresis have shown

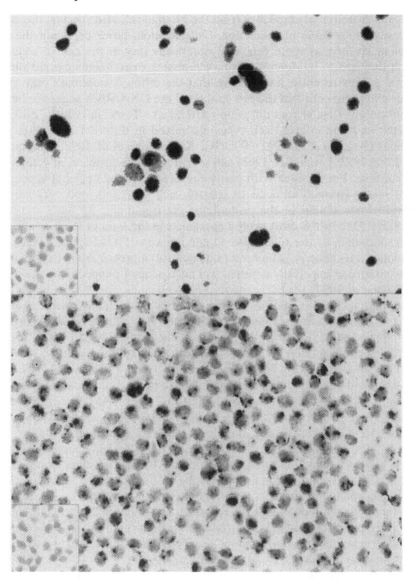

Fig. 10.1. (a) *In situ* PCR and (b) CARD–Nanogold–silver ISH performed on cytospinned and formalin post-fixed SiHa cells. This cervical carcinoma cell line is known to contain 1–2 copies of HPV 16 DNA (human papillomavirus type 16). after amplification of a relevant DNA sequence during *in situ* PCR and subsequent detection by Nanogold–silver ISH, the whole nuclei are filled with DNA product, which after detection gives a masked black appearance of these structures (a). CARD–Nanogold–silver ISH on the other hand yields punctate, spotty staining of the sites containing the single virus copies (b). The size of the spot obtained depends on the concentration of biotinylated tyramides used. Both preparations are counterstained with eosin. The corresponding negative controls, counterstained with hematoxylin, are shown as inserts.

183

that 'out-diffusion' of amplicons from the original cell often occurs; this is not an easily controllable phenomenon. Out-diffusion, however, is not the real problem, as long as some (enough) amplicons stay in the cell of origin in which they are to be detected. But, cell-mixing experiments carried out by several groups recently, have shown that the diffused amplicons may afterwards enter into cells that did not contained the DNA/RNA sequence before amplification ('back/cross-diffusion' artefacts). Tests in which different infected and non-infected cell types are mixed in different and exact proportions (Bagasra *et al.* 1992, 1995a,b,c; Komminoth *et al.* 1992; Komminoth and Long 1993; Long *et al.* 1993) can reveal the same problem in cytological preparations. For sections, with partly cut surfaces of the nuclei, it appears to be at least extremely difficult to control such processes, and very careful, individual adjustment of the proteolytoc pre-treatments for each section is necessary. One of the most skillful specialists in the field of IS-PCR and one of the founders of the technique, Omar Bagasra (Philadelphia, USA), has developed a technique that allows exact control of proteinase K treatment by visual control in a specially adjusted wet microscope ('peppery Bagasra dots') (Bagasra *et al.* 1994).

Another technique, developed by us, is *in situ* self-sustained sequence replication-based amplification (*in situ* 3SR, IS-3SR) (Zehbe *et al.* 1994a). We have applied the 3SR principle (Gingeras *et al.* 1990a,b,) successfully for the *in situ* detection of RNA for the first time. In the meantime, another research team has also applied the 3SR principle *in situ* (Höfler *et al.* 1995). The technique is based on a reiterated cycling of reverse transcription and transcription reactions catalysed by avian myeloblastosis virus (AMV) reverse transcriptase and T7 RNA polymerase, respectively, to replicate an RNA target via RNA/DNA hybrids and double-stranded cDNA intermediates. The cDNA of the original RNA contains a phage (T7) RNA polymerase promoter that is used as a template for an approximately 10^7-fold amplification within 1 to 2 h under favourable conditions. Owing to the action of *Escherichia coli* RNase H, which only destroys the RNA or RNA/DNA hybrids, denaturation steps are not required. IS-3SR, therefore, does not require expensive, special instrumentation. However, it is a relatively complicated set-up, with numerous steps involving time-consuming specificity tests and expensive reagents. Therefore, we did not develop this technique, further.

To date, as can be deduced from the above discussion, no consensus has been reached regarding IS-PCR. We presently recommend the use of IS-PCR for research purposes only. Numerous specificity tests, which are both expensive and time-consuming, have to be included in all experiments, and protocols are still under development. Some authors still claim that IS-PCR is already a routine and rapid detection method of low copy RNA (and DNA) (Nuovo 1996a), but regret that the technique 'demands some skill' (Nuovo 1996b). In our experience, and from personal communication with a number of other scientists using the technique, IS-PCR as available at present must be regarded as relatively unreliable, complicated, and expensive. Only if the conditions are perfect, is single copy DNA or RNA detection possible. Even with the most dedicated (and costly) equipment for IS-PCR available today, reproducibility is still far from 100%. Therefore, instead of presenting intermediate cookbook recipes, we will, in the following section, suggest highly sensitive alternatives of molecular morphological techniques able to detect single copies of DNA, and probably also RNA, in routinely formalin-fixed and paraffin-embedded specimens, and in cytology.

Nanogold–silver *in situ* hybridization

The detection sensitivity of ISH depends to a high degree on the system used for detection of the probe. Enzyme-based, streptavidin–biotin methods, utilizing non-radioactive reporter molecules as probe label (biotin, digoxigenin, etc.; for review see Chevalier *et al.* 1997), followed by peroxidase–diaminobenzidine–H_2O_2 or alkaline phosphatase–nitroblue tetrazolium systems, are in widespread use, and numerous protocols for the detection of hybridization sites based on fluorescence ISH (FISH) have been published (see this book and, for example, Giaid *et al.* 1989; Chan and McGee 1990; Höfler 1990; Herrington and McGee 1992; Luke *et al.* 1997; Paragas *et al.* 1997). A number of papers deal with the use of gold as the label for ISH (Varndell *et al.* 1984; Gu *et al.* 1988; Jackson *et al.* 1990; Troxler *et al.* 1990; Zehbe *et al.* 1992b, 1993a, 1994a,b,c, 1995, 1997; Hacker *et al.* 1993, 1994, 1995, 1996a,b,c, 1997' DeBault and Wang 1994; Hacker and Danscher 1994; Aliviatos *et al.* 1996; Powel *et al.* 1997). Enzyme- and fluorescent-based ISH detection methods have several disadvantages compared with the more delicate, particulate IGSS methods. FITC- and alkaline phosphatase-based systems are regarded as non-permanent stainings and the disadvantages include the fading of most fluorescent labels, the need for an expensive fluorescence microscope, the alcohol solubility of some peroxidase and alkaline phosphatase stains, and false-positive results in combination with prolonged NBT/BCIP development. Peroxidase-based techniques appear to give less spatial resolution than IGSS. Application of IGSS-ISH, if carried out by experienced laboratory technicians aware of the special precautions needed for every kind of silver technique (using only carefully cleaned glassware and ultrapure water for all solutions) gives black staining of positive structures, which stand out distinctly against the unlabelled background tissue. The subsequent transfer of LM sections to the EM may then also allow sublocalization of specific nucleic acid sequences to intracellular compartments, e.g. virus-infected cells at the ultrastructural level (the 'pop-off technique', of W. Muss in Zehbe *et al.* 1993 in Hacker *et al* 1996).

Nanogold–silver ISH is a highly sensitive, alternative, low cost, and rapid method for routine use, the histopathology laboratory (Figs 10.2 and 10.3). It is based on silver amplification of a novel reagent, *Nanogold*^{TM}, covalently

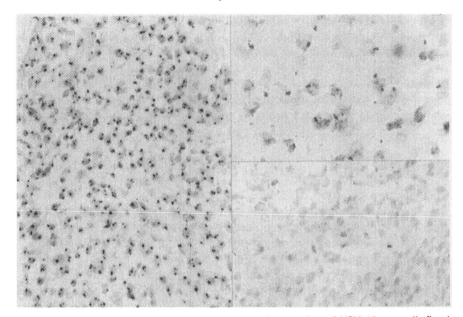

Fig. 10.2. Cervical carcinoma containing one or a few copies of HPV 16 per cell, fixed overnight at room temperature in neutral phosphate-buffered 4% paraformaldehyde solution and paraffin embedded. 4 μm sections mounted on silanized glass slides were stained *in situ* with the CARD–Nanogold–silver ISH technique (a) and showed relatively large single spots in each tumour cell. The straightforward Nanogold–silver ISH technique (without CARD amplification) showed very small single spots which can only be seen in high power magnification (b) The specificity control, in which the DNA probe during the actual hybridization is replaced by pure buffers, showed no specific staining (c). Owing to the extremely high amplification used in the detection procedure, a few tiny silver precipitates are also seen. This case was rated negative when a conventional streptavidin–peroxidase–DAB system or a conventional streptavidin–alkaline phosphatase–NBT/BCIP ISH system was used.

bound to streptavidin (Nanoprobes, Stony Brook, NY). For many years investigators had used colloidal gold as a marker, which is a clump of gold atoms formed by reduction of gold ions in solution to a sphere of gold metal. Adsorption of antibodies to colloidal gold was first described by Faulk and Taylor (1971) and led to many important applications in medicine and biology. Streptavidin may also be adsorbed to colloidal gold, but its performance was reported to be poor for ISH detection (Troxler *et al.* 1990). Although colloidal gold has worked in many applications, a number of practical limitations have been noted.

1. The relatively large size (>4 nm) of colloidal gold, or aggregation in even 1 nm colloidal gold conjugates, limits penetration into cells, giving poor detection in such cases (Vandré and Burry 1992; Robinson and Takizawa, 1996).

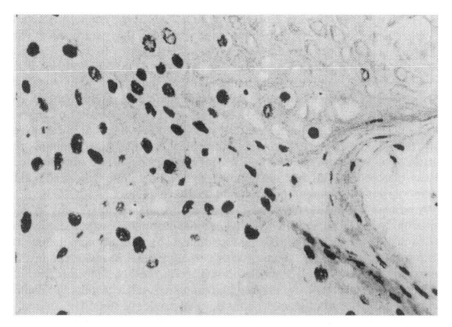

Fig. 10.3. Condyloma acuminatum prepared as in Fig. 10.2, stained with the straight-forward Nanogold–silver ISH technique (without CARD amplification). Large numbers of black-labelled epithelial nuclei harbouring HPV 6/11 were obtained, distinctly standing out against the eosin and Nuclear Fast Red-counterstained background. Serial sections of this case were stained with conventional streptavidin–peroxidase ISH and showed faintly stained nuclei, which were smaller in number than those obtained with Nanogold–silver ISH.

2. Since molecules are only adsorbed to colloidal gold, and not covalently bound, they are been found to 'fall off' to some extent, with time (Horisberger and Clerc 1985), a fact that can further hinder an experiment by allowing the freed antibody or streptavidin to bind to target sites and thereby reduce sensitivity (Kramarcy and Sealock 1990).

3. Colloidal gold conjugates can aggregate, again reducing performance when penetration is involved (Hainfeld 1990; Vandré and Burry 1992).

4. Owing to phenomena that are not yet understood, possibly related to the charge of colloidal gold, limitations are found when detecting intranuclear substances. Reduced labelling is found, for example, in immuno-cytochemistry when staining for Ki-67 or steroid receptors, and also in ISH for intranuclear DNA (G.W. Hacker, unpublished observations).

A different approach is to use gold compounds. An undecagold cluster had already been described in by McPartlin *et al.* (1969). This cluster has only 11 gold atoms in a 0.82 nm core, with the surface gold atoms being covalently attached to phosphorus atoms, and with organic groups on the outside. It may be synthesized with a single reactive group, such as an amine, maleimide (which reacts with thiols), or *N*-hydroxysuccinimide ester (which reacts with amines). This provides a way to couple the gold covalently to the molecule to be tagged in a stable and predictable way (Hainfeld 1987). These conjugates have been found to retain their initial activity even after a year. A similar larger gold cluster ('Nanogold') containing *c*.67 cold atoms (the X-ray structure has not yet been solved) in a 1.4 nm core was made to improve visibility (Hainfeld and Furuja 1992). It was found that this cluster developed silver far better than the 11-gold atom cluster, while still retaining the advantageous properties of stable covalent bonding, small size (for enhanced tissue penetration and high resolution), and good solution properties that inhibit aggregation, adsorption, and non-specific binding.

A number of investigators have now found Nanogold to be substantially superior to colloidal gold in cytological and histological studies, even by electron microscopy (EM). It was also found to penetrate into tissues by 40 μm (Sun *et al.* 1995). Demonstrating its usefulness to make conjugates, probably outside of the realm of colloidal gold, the 11-amino acid peptide substance, P, was covalently coupled and found to localize just as ^{125}I-labelled peptide did. The gold-labelled substance P could be followed on poly-acrylamide gels using silver amplification (autometallography), and its targeting to neural tissue could be competed off with unlabelled substance P (Segond von Banchet and Heppelmann 1995). Other newer developments include: the information of Nanogold coupled to fluorescent molecules (and an antibody or streptavidin) so that localization may be followed by fluor-escence, conventional transmission light microscopy (LM), and also by EM in the same experiment (Powell *et al.* 1997; Robinson and Vandré 1997); the formation of gold lipids (Hainfeld 1996); and Nanogold–DNA conjugates (Alivisatos *et al.* 1996; Malecki 1996). Nanogold–streptavidin conjugates are made by reacting a mono-*N*-hydroxysuccinimide ester of Nanogold with amino groups of streptavidin. The reaction is controlled to yield 1–2 Nanogold particles per streptavidin (a tetrameric protein). The product is purified by gel filtration chromatography to isolate the desired single streptavidin (tetramer) with gold attached, which is separated cleanly from any protein aggregates or free Nanogold. This well-defined and purified product has excellent penetration properties, and since there are four biotin-binding sites per streptavidin, its activity is not impaired by the one or two small gold particles bound per molecule.

In the Nanogold–silver ISH set-up proposed by us, streptavidin–Nanogold is used to detect biotin without a bridging antibody, or to detect FITC or digoxigenin indirectly with a link by a biotinylated specific antibody. Silver amplification is done with silver acetate autometallography (Hacker *et al.* 1988; Danscher *et al.* 1993, 1995). Primarily, we used this new system with great success for IS-PCR, but subsequently determined that its separate use without PCR amplification also gives a very high sensitivity, near to the single copy level (Hacker *et al.* 1996b, 1977). Nanogold–silver ISH turned out to be an elegant and rapid way to overcome the threshold limit for detection of biotinylated probes, which in combination with peroxidase as the label, had been calculated at about 20 copies per cell (Zehbe *et al.* 1992a). Sometimes we even observed spot-like reactions in SiHa cells, which are known to contain only one copy of HPV 16 DNA per cell (Friedl *et al* 1970), but this was not always reproducible. Streptavidin–Nanogold combined with highly stringent ISH protocols (patent pending) gave high versatility and sensitivity (Hacker *et al.* 1996a,b, 1997) and can be completed within about 4 h. It therefore appears to be an ideal method for fast and reliable routine use. Excellent labelling properties and distinctly black stains were obtained, which were superior to previous procedures. Cervical carcinomas with very few HPV 16 copies per cell showed up as punctate, spotty staining inside the tumour cell nuclei (Fig. 10.2) (Hacker *et al.* 1997). Other DNA viruses tested included various other types of HPV, cytomegalovirus (CMV), Epstein–Barr virus (EBV), herpes simplex virus (HSV), and adenivorus type V. The morphology was far better than that obtained with IS-PCR. Experiments employing standard ISH methods (peroxidase–DAB and alkaline phosphatase–NBT/BCIP kits, Enzo, New York, USA) on serial sections of Nanogold–silver ISH-stained condylomas have shown that Nanogold ISH, in most cases, gave numbers of infected cells comparable to those detected with the other systems tested, but with staining of higher contrast. In addition, a number of cases clearly demonstrated a higher sensitivity of Nanogold–silver ISH: Nanogold–silver ISH was sometimes also positive on cases that tested negative with both of the other techniques used. ISH kits with streptavidin–Nanogold optimized for supersensitive, reliable and easy to perform nucleic acid detection are now commercially available (Nanoprobes, Stony Brook, NY; see also Internet web site <www.nanoprobes.com>).

CARD–Nanogold–silver *in situ* hybridization

A number of systems have been developed for supersensitive ISH without the necessity for amplification of nucleic acids, as is done in IS-PCR or IS-3SR (e.g. Macechko *et al.* 1997; Paragas *et al.* 1997; Schmidt *et al.* 1997; Van Gijlswijk *et al.* 1997; Tbakhi *et al.* 1998; Totos *et al.* submitted). Instead, these new systems use label amplification rather than DNA amplification. The CARD technology (catalysed reporter deposition), commercialized under the term tyramide signal amplification (TSA™, TSA-indirect (ISH) kit, code NEL 730 A; NEN Life Sciences Products, Boston, USA) was originally developed by Bobrow *et al.* (1989). Today, real CARD appears to be a breakthrough technology which can make non-radioactive ISH techniques the preferred choice over IS-PCR and related technologies. It allows for a broad range of fluorescence and chromogenic detection, and provides significantly increased sensitivity and increased spatial resolution (Kerstens *et al.* 1995; Hacker *et al.* 1996a,b, 1997; Macechko *et al.* 1997; Schmidt *et al.* 1997; Van Gijlswijk *et al.* 1997; Zehbe *et al.* 1997; Tbakhi *et al.* submitted; Totos *et al.* submitted).

Very recently, we combined CARD with Nanogold–silver ISH (Fig. 10.4) (Hacker *et al.* 1996a,b, 1997; Zehbe *et al.* 1997; Tubbs *et al.* 1997a,b; Tbakhi *et al.* submitted; Totos *et al* submitted). Using this specific set-up, single gene copy sensitivity was obtained in a DNA-labelling system (Hacker *et al.* 1997; Zehbe *et al.* 1997) (Fig. 10.1). IS-PCR yields similar sensitivity, but usually masks and compromises morphological detail (Fig. 10.1) and may produce spurious results owing to amplicon diffusion or other mechanisms. Compared with IS-PCR, the likelihood of false-positive results is greatly reduced.

In CARD, biotinylated tyramide (BT reagent) is deposited at peroxidase-labelled sites (Fig. 10.4). In the first step, specific ISH is carried out using biotinylated, FITC-labelled, or digoxigenin-labelled probes. The reporter molecule is primarily detected either directly with streptavidin–peroxidase, or indirectly using an antibody to the reporter molecule (e.g. anti-FITC or anti-digoxigenin) as a link to streptavidin–peroxidase. Each of the peroxidase molecules labelling the ISH sites in a tree-like manner is a target for a number of biotin-labelled tyramide (BT) molecules. This multiplication of reporter molecule sites leads to numerous biotin molecules being available for the next detection step, which is carried out by streptavidin–Nanogold. Subsequent silver amplification with silver acetate or silver lactate autometallography (Danscher 1981a,b, 1984; Hacker *et al.* 1988; Danscher *et al.* 1993, 1995) makes the accumulation of Nanogold label easily visible in the LM and EM. It has been found that the labelling density, and therefore the sensitivity, is greater when higher concentrations of BT reagent are used. At the same time, as seen in EM studies, the BT–Nanogold 'tree' is growing, and the distance of the gold particles from the original hybridization site also becomes greater (C. Schöfer, Vienna, personal communication). In the LM, this is seen as an increasingly larger spot of gold–silver staining.

The novel CARD–Nanogold–silver ISH gave, for the first time, single gene copy sensitivity for both DNA (Fig. 10.1) (Hacker *et al.* 1997; Zehbe *et al.* 1997) and, probably, RNA (Fig. 10.5) (Tubbs, in Hacker *et al.* 1997) in cyto-logical material, as well as in histological sections from formalin-fixed paraffin-embedded SiHa cells. Compared with conventional standard tech-niques (peroxidase–DAB and alkaline phosphatase–NBT/BCIP kits, Enzo, New York, USA), far superior results were frequently obtained (Hacker *et al.* 1997). The appearance of the staining in SiHa cells known to contain only one or a few copies of HPV type 16 DNA was a spotty, punctate black labelling (Fig. 10.1) (Hacker *et al.* 1997; Tubbs *et al.* 1997a; Zehbe *et al.* 1997). A series of cervical carcinomas showed positive HPV 16 detection in nearly 100% of cases (Fig. 10.2) (Hacker *et al.* 1997; Zehbe *et al.* 1997). ISH tests also included a series of other types of DNA viruses, all of which also gave reliable results.

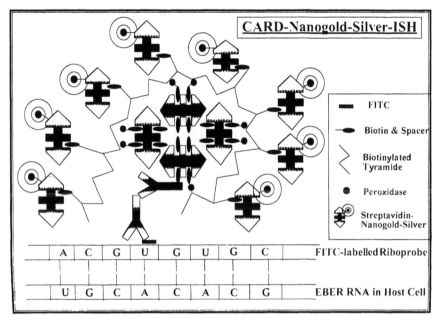

Fig. 10.4. Schematic representation of the CARD–Nanogold–silver ISH technology. This example shows the detection of EBER RNA from Epstein–Barr virus (EBV) which is hybridized to a FITC-labelled riboprobe. FITC used as the reporter molecule is then immunologically labelled using a specific antibody to FITC, followed by a biotinylated secondary antibody against Ig of the species in which the primary antibody was produced. In the next step, a peroxidase-labelled streptavidin–biotin complex (S-ABC) is bound to the biotin of the second antibody. A number of S-ABC molecules can bind in this way, but for simplicity, only four such S-ABC–peroxidase molecules are included in the figure. This reaction is followed by the real amplification step, in which a huge amount of biotinylated tyramides are precipitated at peroxidase-labelled sites. Finally, Nanogold-labelled streptavidin binds on the 'multiplied' biotin molecules, and silver acetate autometallography amplifies the tiny (1.4 nm) gold particles to sizes visible in the light and electron microscope.

RNA ISH, extensively tested with EBER RNA of Epstein–Barr virus (EBV), and a few experiments so far with mRNA of kappa light chains, gave distinct and sensitive RNA staining (Fig. 10.5). A member of our team, Prof. Raymond Tubbs (Cleveland, OH) has been successful in employing the CARD technology in combination with alkaline phosphatase and with Nanogold–silver ISH on an automated ISH staining machine (Ventana Gen II; Tucson, AR, USA) (Tubbs *et al.* 1997b; Tbakhi *et al.* 1998; Totos *et al.*, submitted). This implementation allows the whole procedure to be performed within only 5 h, which will help greatly in the introduction of CARD technology into routine diagnostic procedures.

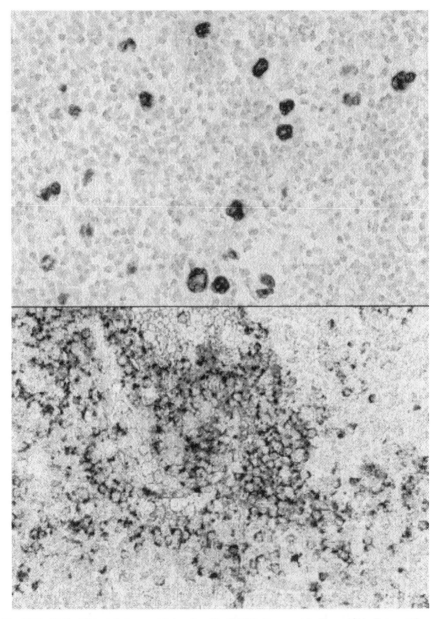

Fig. 10.5. RNA ISH stainings obtained with CARD–Nanogold–silver ISH. Preparations were processed identically to those of Fig. 10.2. EBER RNA of Epstein–Barr virus (EBV) in infected lymphatic tissue was distinctly labelled (a), as was mRNA of kappa light chains in a case of a malignant lymphoma (b).

Conclusions

The CARD technology is a welcome step in the goal of replacing the more costly and unreliable IS-PCR technology. In the *Appendix*, protocols for supersensitive DNA and RNA detection currently used in our laboratories are suggested. As this is a new and still emerging technology, the procedures given should be understood to be guidelines only. The possibility for unwanted deviations from the wanted outcome is still relatively large. This is especially so because the quality of the TSA reagent available does not appear to be consistent yet. Also, a number of variables that are not easily controllable can lead to uneven results. These, to a great extent, include the exactness of the protease pre-treatment used (for supersensitivity, a prolonged proteinase K treatment is necessary, which decreases the survival of morphological details) and the degree of stringency used in the washes following the hybridization step.

Acknowledgements

For joint collaboration in ISH and IS-PCR-related projects, we want to express our sincere thanks to Drs James Hainfeld (Stony Brook, NY, USA), Huici Su (Xi'an, PR China, and Aarhus, Denmark), Greg Totos (visiting international scholar at Cleveland Clinic, OH, USA), Heidi Aichhorn, Cornelia Hauser-Kronberger, Wolfgang H. Muss, Angelika Schiechl, and Elke Zipperer (Salzburg, Austria). We would also like to thank Drs Mark Bobrow, Karl Adler, and Pat Mayer (NEN Life Sciences Products, Boston, MA) and to Dr James Hainfeld again (Nanoprobes, Stony Brook, NY, USA) for providing the excellent reagents used in this study.

References

Alivisatos, A.P., Johnsson, J.P., Pink, X., Wilson, T.E., Loweth, C.J., Bruchez, M.P., Jr, and Schultz, P.G. (1996). Organization of 'nanocrystal molecules' using DNA. *Nature*, **382**, 609–11.

Bagasra, O. (1990). Polymerase chain reaction *in situ*. (editorial note). *Amplifications* March, 20–21.

Bagasra, O., Hauptman, S.P., Lischner, H.W., Sachs, M., and Pomerantz, R.J. (1992). Detection of HIV-1 provirus in mononuclear cells by *in situ* PCR. *N. Engl. J. Med.*, **326**, 1385–91.

Bagasra, O., Seshamma, T., Hansen, J., Bobroski, L., Saikumari, P., Pestaner, J.P., and Pomerantz, R.J. (1994). Application of *in situ* PCR methods in molecular biology: I. Details of methodology for general use. *Cell Vision*, **1**, 324–35.

Bagasra, O., Hui, Z., Bobroski, L., Seshamma, T., Saikumari, P., and Pomerantz, R.J. (1995a). One step amplification of HIV-1 mRNA and DNA at a single cell level by *in situ* polymerase chain reaction. *Cell Vision*, **2**, 425–9.

193

In situ *Hybridization*

Bagasra, O., Michaels, F., Mu, Y., Bobroski, L., Spitsin, S.V., Fu, Z.F., and Koprowski, H. (1995b). Activation of the inducible form of nitric oxide synthetase in the brains of patients with multiple sclerosis. *Proc. Natl. Acad. Sci. USA*, **92**, 12041–5.

Bagasra, O., Seshamma, T., Hansen, J., Bobroski, L., Saikumari, P., and Pomerantz, R.J. (1995c). Application of *in situ* PCR methods in molecular biology: II. Special applications in electron microscopy, cytogenetics and immunohistochemistry. *Cell Vision*, **2**, 61–70.

Bagasra, O., Bobroski, L.E., Pestaner, J.P., Seshamma, T., and Pomerantz, R.J. (1996). Localization of HIV-1 in cardiac tissue utilizing *in situ* PCR. *Cell Vision*, **3**, 6–10.

Bobrow, M.N., Thomas, D., Harris, D., Shaughnessy, K.J., and Litt, G.J. (1989). Catalyzed reporter deposition, a novel method of signal amplification. Application to immunoassays. *J. Immunol. Meth.*, **125**, 279–85.

Bobrow, M.N., Shaughnessy, K.J., and Litt, G.J. (1991). Catalyzed reporter deposition a novel method of signal amplification. II. Application to membrane immunoassays. *J. Immunol. Meth.*, **137**, 103–12.

Chan, V.T.-W. and McGee, J.O'D. (1990). Non-radioactive probes: preparation, characterization, and detection. In: *In situ* hybridization: principles and practice, (1st edn), (ed. J.M. Polak and J.O'D McGee), pp. 59–70. Oxford University Press, Oxford.

Chevailer, J., Yi, J., Michel, O., and Tang, X.-M. (1997). Biotin and digoxigenin as labels for light and electron microscopy *in situ* hybridization probes: Where do we stand? *J. Histochem. Cytochem.*, **45**, 481–91.

Chiu, K.P., Cohen, S.H., Morris, D.W., and Jordan, G.W. (1992). Intracellular amplification of proviral DNA in tissue sections using the polymerase chain reaction. *J. Histochem. Cytochem.*, **40**, 333–41.

Danscher, G. (1981a). Histochemical demonstration of heavy metals. A revised version of the sulphide silver method suitable for both light and electron microscopy. *Histochemistry*, **71**, 1–16.

Danscher, G. (1981b). Localization of gold in biological tissue. A photochemical method for light and electronmicroscopy. *Histochemistry*, **71**, 81–8.

Danscher, G. (1984). Autometallography. A new technique for light and electron microscopical visualization of metals in biological tissue (gold, silver, metal sulphides and metal selenides). *Histochemistry*, **81**, 331–5.

Danscher, G. and Norgaard, J.O. (1983). Light microscopic visualization of colloidal gold on resin-embedded tissue. *J. Histochem. Cytochem.*, **31**, 1394–8.

Danscher, G., Hacker, G.W., Norgaard, J.O., and Grimelius, L. (1993). Autometallographic silver amplification of colloidal gold. *J. Histotechnol.*, **16**, 201–7.

Danscher, G., Hacker, G.W., Hauser-Kronberger, C., and Grimelius, L. (1995). Trends in autometallographic silver amplification of colloidal gold particles. In: *Immunogold–silver staining: methods and applications*, (ed. M.A. Hayat), pp. 11–18. CRC Press, Boca Raton.

De Bault, L.E. and Wang, B.-L. (1994). Localization of mRNA by *in situ* transcription and immunogold-silver staining. *Cell Vision*, **1**, 67–70.

Faulk, W.P. and Taylor, G.M. (1971). An immunocolloid method for the electron microscope. *Immunochemistry*, **8**, 1081–3.

Friedl, F., Kimura, I., Osato, T., and Ito, Y. (1970). Studies on a new human cell line (SiHa) derived from carcinoma of uterus. 1. Its establishment and morphology. *PSEBM*, **135**, 543–5.

Giaid, A., Hamid, Q., Adams, C., Springall, D.R., Terenghi, G., and Polak, J.M. (1989). Non-isotopic RNA probes. Comparison between different labels and detection systems. *Histochemistry*, **93**, 191–6.

Gingeras, T.R., Whitfield, K.M., and Kwoh, D.Y. (1990a). Unique features of the self-sustained sequence replication (3SR) reaction in the *in vitro* amplification of nucleic acids. *Ann. Biol. Clin.*, **48**, 498–501.

Gingeras, T.R., Richman, D.D., Kwoh, D.Y., and Guatelli, J.C. (1990b). Methodologies for in vitro nucleic acid amplification and their applications. *Vet. Microbiol.*, **24**, 235–51.

Gu, J. (1994). Principles and applications of *in situ* PCR. *Cell Vision*, **1**, 8–19.

Gu, J., Linnoila, R.I., Saibel, N.L., Gazdar, A.F., Minna Brooks, B.J., Hollis, G.F., and Kirsch, I.R. (1988). A study of myc-related gene expression in small cell lung cancer by *in situ* hybridization. *Am. J. Pathol.*, **132**, 13–17.

Haase, A.T., Retzel, E.F., and Staskus, K.A. (1990). Amplification and detection of lentiviral DNA inside cells. *Proc. Natl. Acad. Sci. USA*, **87**, 4971–5.

Hacker, G.W. and Danscher, G. (1994). Recent advances in immunogold–silver staining—autometallography. *Cell Vision*, **1**, 102–9.

Hacker, G.W., Grimelius, L., Danscher, G., Bernatzky, G., Muss, W., Adam, H., and Thurner, J. (1988). Silver acetate autometallography: an alternative enhancement technique for immunogold–silver staining (IGSS) and silver amplification of gold, silver, mercury and zinc in tissues. *J. Histotechnol.*, **11**, 213–21.

Hacker, G.W., Graf, A.-H., Hauser-Kronberger, C., Wirnsberger, G., Schiechl, A., Bernatzky, G., Wittauer, U., Su, H., Adam, H., Thurner, J., Danscher, G., and Grimelius, L. (1993). Application of silver acetate autometallography and gold–silver staining methods for *in situ* DNA hybridization. *Chinese Med. J.*, **106**, 83–92.

Hacker, G.W., Zehbe, I., Hauser-Kronberger, C., Gu, J., Graf, A.-H., and Deitze, O. (1994). *In situ* detection of DNA and mRNA sequences by immunogold–silver staining (IGSS). *Cell Vision*, **1**, 30–7.

Hacker, G.W., Danscher, G., Grimelius, L., Hauser-Kronberger, C., Muss, W.H., Schiechl, A., Gu, J., and Dietze, O. (1995). Silver staining techniques, with special reference to the use of different silver salts in light and electron microscopical immunogold–silver staining. In: *Immunogold–silver staining: methods and applications*, (ed. M.A. Hayat) pp. 20–45. CRC Press, Boca Raton.

Hacker, G.W., Zehbe, I., Hainfeld, J., Sällström, J., Hauser-Kronberger, C., Graf, A.-H., Su, H., Dietze, O., and Bagasra, O. (1996a). High-performance Nanogold *in situ* hybridization and *in situ* PCR. *Cell Vision*, **3**, 209–14.

Hacker, G.W., Zehbe, I., Hainfeld, J., Graf, A.-H., Hauser-Kronberger, C., Schiechl, A., Su, H., and Dietze, O. (1996b). High performance Nanogold-*in situ* hybridization and its use in the detection of hybridized and PCR amplified microscopical preparations. In: *Microscopy and Microanalysis 1996, Proceedings of the Microscopical Society of America, Minneapolis, Minnesota*, (ed. G.W. Bailey, J.M. Corbett, R.V.W. Dimlich, J.R. Michael, and N.J. Zaluzec) San Francisco Press, San Francisco.

Hacker, G.W., Muss, W.H., Hauser-Kronberger, C., Danscher, G., Rufner, R., Gu, J., Su, H., Andreasen, A., Stoltenberg, M., and Dietze, O. (1996c). Electron microscopical autometallography: immunogold–silver staining (IGSS) and heavy-metal-histochemistry. *Methods* (Companion *Meth. Enzymol.*), **10**, 257–69.

Hacker, G.W., Hauser-Kronberger, C., Zehbe, I., Su, H., Schiechl, A., Dietze, O., and

In situ *Hybridization*

Tubbs, R. (1997). *In situ* localization of DNA and RNA sequences: super-sensitive *in situ* hybridization using streptavidin–Nanogold–silver staining: minireview, protocols and possible applications. *Cell Vision*, **4**, 54–65.

Hainfeld, J.F. (1987). A small gold-conjugated antibody label: improved resolution for electron microscopy. *Science*, **236**, 450–3.

Hainfeld, J.F. (1990). STEM analysis of Janssen Autoprobe One. In: *Proc. XIIth Int. Cong. Elec. Microsc.* (ed. G.W. Bailey), pp. 954–5. San Francisco Press, San Francisco.

Hainfeld, J.F. and Furuja, F.R. (1992). A 1.4-nm gold cluser covalently attached to antibodies improves immunolabeling. *J. Histochem. Cytochem.*, **30**, 177–84.

Herrington, C.S. and McGee, J.O'D. (ed.) (1992). *Diagnostic molecular pathology. A practical approach, Vols I and II.* Oxford University Press, Oxford.

Höfler, H. (1990). Principles of in situ hybridization. In: *In situ hybridization: principles and practice,* (1st edn), (ed. J.M. Polak and J.O'D. McGee), pp. 15–29. Oxford University Press, Oxford.

Höfler, H., Pütz, B., Mueller, J.D., Neubert, W., Sutter, G., and Gais, P. (1995). Methods in laboratory investigation: *in situ* amplification of measles virus RNA by the self-sustained sequence replication reaction. *Lab. Invest.*, **73**, 577–85.

Holgate, C.S., Jackson, P., Cowen, P.N., and Bird, C.C. (1983). Immunogold–silver staining: new method of immunostaining with enhanced sensitivity. *J. Histochem. Cytochem.*, **31**, 938–94.

Horisberger, M. and Clerc, M.F. (1985). Labelling of colloidal gold with protein A. A quantitative study. *Histochemistry*, **82**, 219.

Jackson, P., Dockey, D.A., Lewis, F.A., and Wells, M. (1990). Application of 1 nm gold probes on paraffin wax sections for *in situ* hybridisation histochemistry. *J. Clin. Pathol.*, **43**, 810–12.

Kerstens, H.M., Poddighe, P.J., and Hanselaar, A.G. (1995). A novel *in situ* hybridization signal amplification method based on the deposition of biotinylated tyramine. *J. Histochem. Cytochem.*, **43**, 347–52.

Komminoth, P. and Long, A.A. (1993). *In situ* polymerase chain reaction. An overview of methods, applications and limitations of a new molecular technique. *Virch. Arch. B Cell Pathol.*, **64**, 67–73.

Komminoth, P., Long, A., Ray, R., and Wolfe, H.J. (1992). *In situ* polymerase chain reaction detection of viral DNA, single-copy genes, and gene rearrangements in cell suspensions and cytosprins. *Diagn. Mol. Pathol.*, **1**, 85–97.

Kramarcy, N.R. and Sealock, R. (1990). Commercial preparations of colloidal gold-antibody complexes frequently contain free active antibody. *J. Histochem. Cytochem.*, **39**, 37–9.

Long, A.A., Komminoth, P., Lee, E., and Wolfe, H.J. (1993). Comparison of indirect and direct *in-situ* polymerase, chain reaction in cell preparations and tissue sections. *Histochemistry*m **99**, 151–62.

Luke, S., Varkey, J.A., Belogolovkin, V., and Ladoulis, C.T. (1997). Current state of fluorescence *in situ* hybridization (FISH) in diagnostic pathology. *Cell Vision*, **4**, 16–31.

Macechko, P.T., Krueger, L., Hirsch, B., and Erlandsen, S.L. (1997). Comparison of immunologic amplification vs enzymatic deposition of fluorochrome-conjugated tyramide as detection systems for FISH. *J. Histochem. Cytochem.*, **45**, 359–63.

Malecki, M. (1996). Energy filtering transmission electron microscopy of transfected

DNA. In: *Proceedings Microscopy and Microanalysis*, (ed. G.W. Bailey, J.M. Corbett, R.V.W. Dimlich, J.R. Michael, and N.J. Zaluzec, pp. 924–5. San Francisco Press, San Francisco.

Martinez, A., Miller, M.J., Catt, K.J., and Cuttitta, F. (1997). Adrenomedullin receptor expression in human lung and in pulmonary tumors. *J. Histochem. Cytochem.*, **45**, 159–64.

McPartlin, M., Mason, R., and Malatesta, I. (1969). Novel cluster complexes of gold(0)–gold(1). *J. Chem. Soc. Chem. Commun.*, 334.

Nuovo, G.J. (1991). Detection of human papillomavirus DNA in formalin-fixed tissues by *in situ* hybridization after amplification by polymerase chain reaction. *Am. J. Pathol.*, **139**, 847–54.

Nuovo, G.J. (1992). *PCR in situ hybridization*. Raven Press, New York.

Nuovo, G.J. (1996a). The foundations of successful RT *in situ* PCR. *Front. Biosci.*, **1**, C4–C15.

Nuovo, G.J. (1996b). Detection of viral infections by *in situ* PCR: theoretical considerations and possible value in diagnostic pathology. *J. Clin. Lab. Anal.*, **10**, 335–49.

Nuovo, G.J., Gallery, F., MacConnell, P., Becker, J., and Bloch, W. (1991). An improved technique for the *in situ* detection of DNA after polymerase chain reaction amplification. *Am. J. Pathol.*, **139**, 1239–44.

Paragas, V.B., Zhang, Y-Z., Haughland, R.P., and Singer, V.L. (1997). The ELF-97 alkaline phosphatase substrate provides a bright, photostable, fluorescent signal amplification method for FISH. *J. Histochem. Cytochem.*, **45**, 345–58.

Polak, J.M., and J.O'D. McGee, J.O'D. (ed.) (1990). *In situ hybridization: principles and practice*, (1st edn). Oxford University Press, Oxford.

Powell, R.D., Halsey, C.M.R., Spector, D.L., Kaurin, S.L., McCann, J., and Hainfeld, J.F. (1997). A covalent fluorescent–gold immunoprobe: simultaneous detection of a pre-mRNA splicing factor by light and electron microscopy. *J. Histochem. Cytochem.*, **45**, 947–56.

Robinson, J.M. and Takizawa, T. (1996). Novel labeling methods for EM analysis of ultrathin cryosections. In: *Proceedings Microscopy and Microanalysis*, (ed. G.W. Bailey, J.M. Corbett, R.V.W. Dimlich, J.R. Michael, and N.J. Zaluzec, pp. 894–5. San Francisco Press, San Francisco.

Robinson, J.M. and Vandrée D.D. (1997). Efficient immunocytochemical labeling of leukocyte microtubules with FluoroNanogold: an important tool for correlative microscopy. *J. Histochem. Cytochem.*, **45**, 631–42.

Sällström, J., Alemi, M., Spets, H., and Zehbe, I. (1994). Nonspecific amplification *in situ* PCR by direct incorporation of reporter molecules. *Cell Vision*, **1**, 243–51.

Schmidt, B.F., Chao, J., Zhi, Z., DeBiasio, R., and Fisher, G. (1997). Signal amplification in the detection of single-copy DNA and RNA by enzyme-catalyzed deposition (CARD) of the novel fluorescent reporter substrate Cy3.29-tyramide. *J. Histochem. Cytochem.*, **45**, 365–373.

Segond von Banchet, G. and Heppelmann, B. (1995). Non-radioactive localization of substance P binding site in rat brain and spinal cord using peptides labeled with 1.4-nm gold particles. *J. Histochem. Cytochem.*, **43**, 821–7.

Springall, D.R., Hacker, G.W., Grimelius, L., and Polak, J.M. (1994). The potential of the immunogold–silver staining method for paraffin sections. *Histochemistry*, **81**, 603–8.

In situ *Hybridization*

Sun, X.J., Tolbert, L.P., and Hildebrand, J.G. (1995). Using laser scanning confocal microscopy as a guide for electron microscopic study: a simple method for correlation of light and electron microscopy. *J. Histochem, Cytochem.*, **43**, 329–35.

Tbakhi, A., Hauser-Kronberger, C., Totos, G., Pettay, J., Baunoch, D., Hacker, G.W., and Tubbs, R.R. (1998). Fixation conditions for DNA and RNA *in situ* hybridization: a reassessment of molecular morphology dogma. *Am. J. Pathol.*, **109**, 16–23.

Totos, G., Pettay, J., Tbakhi, A., Hauser-Kronberger, C., Hacker, G.W., and Tubbs, R.R., Automated kinetic mode detection of single viral gene copy by DNA *in situ* hybridization. *Lab. Invest.*, submitted.

Troxler, M., Pasamontes, L., Egger, D., and Bienz, K. 1990. *In situ* hybridization for light and electron microscopy: a comparison of methods for the localization of viral RNA using bitinylated DNA and RNA probes. *J. Virol. Meth.*, **30**, 1–14.

Tubbs, R., Zehbe, I., Hauser-Kronberger, C., and Hacker, G.W. (1997a). Single HPV gene copy is detectable in paraffin sections of formalin fixed material by the CARD-Nanogold non-isotopic technique. *Mod. Pathol.*, **10**, 135A (also inL: *Lab. Invest.*, **76**, 184A, # 1083).

Tubbs, R., Hacker, G.W., Hauser-Kronberger, C., Zehbe, I., Totos, G., Tbakhi, A., Pettay, J., and Baunoch, D. (1997b). Reappraisal of primary fixation conditions for DNA and RNA *in situ* hybridization. *Mod. Pathol.*, **10**, 184A (also in: *Lab. Invest.*, **76**, 184A, # 1984).

Vandre, D.D. and Burry, R.W. (1992). Immunoelectron microscopic localization of phosphoproteins associated with the mitotic spindle. *J. Histochem. Cytochem.*, **40**, 1837–47.

Van Gijlswijk, R.P.M., Ziklmans, H.J.M.A.A., Wiegant, J., Bobrow, M.N., Erickson, T.J., Adler, K.E., Tanke, H.J., and Raap, A.K. (1997). Fluorochrome-labeled tyramides: use in immunocytochemistry and fluorescence *in situ* hybridization. *J. Histochem. Cytochem.*, **45**, 375–82.

Varndell, I.M., Polak, J.M., Sikri, K.L., Minth, C.D., Bloom, S.R., and Dixon, J.E. (1984). Visualisation of messenger RNA directing peptide synthesis by *in situ* hybridisation using a novel single-stranded cDNA probe. *Histochemistry*, **81**, 597–601.

Zehbe, I., Rylander, E., Strand, A., and Wilander, E. (1992a). *In situ* hybridization for the detection of human papillomavirus (HPV) in gynaecological biopsies. A study of two commercial kits. *Anticancer Res.*, **12**, 1383–8.

Zehbe, I., Hacker, G.W., Sällström, J., Rylander, E., and Wilander, E. (1992b). *In situ* polymerase chain reaction (in situ PCR) combined with immunoperoxidase staining and immunogold-silver staining (IGSS) techniques. Detection of single copies of HPV in SiHa cells. *Anticancer Res.*, **12**, 2165–8.

Zehbe, I., Hacker, G.W., Muss, W.H., Sällström, J., Rylander, E., Graf, A.-H., Prömer, H., and Wilander, E. (1993a). An improved protocol of *in situ* polymerase chain reaction (PCR) for the detection of human papillomavirus (HPV). *J. Cancer Res. Clin. Oncol.*, **119**, (Suppl.), 22.

Zehbe, I., Rylander, E., Strand, A., and Wilander, E. (1993b). Use of probemix and omniprobe biotinylated cDNA probes for detecting HPV infection in biopsy specimens from the genital tract. *J. Clin. Pathol.*, **46**, 437–40.

Zehbe, I., Hacker, G.W., Sällström, J.F., Rylander, E., and Wilander, E. (1994a). Self-sustained sequence replication-based amplification (3SR) for the *in situ* detection of mRNA in cultured cells. *Cell Vision*, **1**, 20–4.

Supersensitive in situ *DNA and RNA localization*

Zehbe, I., Hacker, G.W., Sällström, J.F., Muss, W.H., Hauser-Kronberger, C., Rylander, E., and Wilander, E. (1994b). PCR *in situ* hybridization (PISH) and *in situ* self-sustained sequence replication-based amplification (*in situ* 3SR). *Cell Vision*, **1**, 46–7.

Zehbe, I., Hacker, G.W., Hauser-Kronberger, C., Rylander, E., and Wilander, E. (1994c). Indirect and direct *in situ* PCR for the detection of human papillomavirus. An evaluation of two methods and a double staining technique. *Cell Vision*, **1**, 163–7.

Zehbe, I., Hacker, G.W., Sällström, J.F., Muss, W.H., Hauser-Kronberger, C., and Wilander, E. (1995). *In situ* PCR and enzyme-driven *in situ* amplification (*in situ* 3SR) for the detection of viral DNA and mRNA. *Cell Vision*, **2**, 240–2.

Zehbe, I., Hacker, G.W., Su, H., Hauser-Kronberger, C., Hainfeld, J.F., and Tubbs, R. (1997). Sensitive *in situ* hybridization with catalyzed reporter deposition, strepta-vidin–Nanogold· and silver acetate autometallography. *Am. J. Pathol.*, **150**, 1553–61.

Appendix 10.1

Protocol 1. DNA in situ hybridization with streptavidin–Nanogold and silver acetate autometallography

Practical considerations. This is a robust and reliable technique for routine use. It is intended for biotinylated hybridization probes. Other types of reporter molecules may be demonstrated by application of a biotinylated linking antibody system. The sensitivity of Nanogold–silver ISH depends, to a large degree, on the dilution of streptavidin–Nanogold and the duration of silver development applied. Careful adjustment of the protease predigestion is necessary. In some preparations, some degree of unwanted background staining in connective tissue is obtained. This is in part due to fixation and possible excessive protease treatment, and can often be reduced by application of higher dilutions of streptavidin–Nanogold.

1. Deparaffinize formaldehyde-fixed sections in fresh xylene (2 × 15 min each).

2. Rinse and rehydrate in degraded alcohols and distilled water (2–3 min each).

3. Soak in phosphate buffered saline (PBS, 20 mM, pH 7.6) for 3 min.

4. Permeabilize with 0.3% Triton X-100 in PBS for 10 min.

5. Incubate with 0.03% proteinase K (code no. 1 373 196, stock solution of 18.6 mg/ml, from Boehringer Mannheim, Germany) in PBS at 37 °C for about 8 min. The duration is critical and has to be tested very carefully, depending on tissue, fixation, and other factors.

6. Rinse in PBS for 2 × 4 min.

7. Rinse in 2 changes of distilled water, dehydrate with graded alcohols (50% isopropanol for 2 min. 70% isopropanol for 2 min, and 98% isopropanol 2 × 2 min each) and air dry sections.

8. Prehydrize with 50% deionized formamide and 10% dextran sulfate in 2 × SSC at 50°C for 5 min.

9. Carefully shake off excess pre-hybridization block.

10. Add one drop of biotinylated DNA probe on the section and cover with a small coverslip. Avoid air bubbles.

11. Heat sections on heating block for denaturation of DNA (92–94°C) for 10 min.

12. Incubate in a moist chamber at 37°C overnight (or for at least 2 h).

13. Post-hybridization washes (5 min each): 4 × SSC two changes, 2 × SSC two times, 0.1 ×SSC, 0.05 × SSC, and then distilled water. During the first wash, coverslips will automatically fall off the slide.

14. Put slides into Lugol's iodine solution (Merck, Germany) for 5 min.

15. Wash in tap water and then distilled water.

16. Put into 2.5% sodium thiosulfate, until sections are colourless (usually a few sec). Then wash in tap water for 5 min and distilled water for 2 min.

17. Immerse in PBS (pH 7.6) containing 0.1% fish–gelatin (45% concentrate— code no. G-7765—available from Sigma, Steinheim, Germany) (PBS–gelatin) for 5 min.

18. Incubate sections with straptavidin–Nanogold (Nanoprobes, Stony Brook, USA) diluted 1:200 to 1:500 in PBS pH 7.6 containing 1% BSA at RT for 60 min.

19. Wash in PBS pH 7.6, 2 × 5 min each.

20. Wash in PBS–gelatin pH 7.6 for 5 min.

21. Repeatedly wash in distilled water for at least 10 min altogether, the last 2 rinses in ultrapure water (EM grade).

22. Perform silver acetate autometallography (see Addendum below).

23. Rinse carefully in tap water for at least 3 min. After silver amplification, sections can be counterstained with nuclear Fast Red, dehydrated, and mounted in Permount™ or in DPX™ (BDH Chemicals, UK). Do not use Eukitt.

Solutions

Phosphate-buffered saline (PBS)@ 10 × PBS (Mg^{2+} and Ca2+ free) pH 7.6: 11.36 g Na_2HPO_4, 2.72 g KH_2PO_4, 87.0 g NaCl in 800 ml distilled water. Adjust pH with concentrated NaOH and add distilled water to a final volume of 1 l.

Standard sodium citrate buffer (SSC): 175/32 g NaCl and 88.23 g sodium citrate in 800 ml distilled water. Adjust pH with NaOH to 7.0 and add distilled water to a final volume of 1 l.

Addendum. Silver acetate autometallography

This method (Hacker *et al.* 1988) can be applied for immunocytochemical IGSS, as well as for lectin histochemistry, ISH, IS-PCR, and the detection of metallic gold and silver, and sulfides or selenides of mercury, silver, and zinc.

(a) Solutions A and B should be freshly prepared for every run.
   Solution A. Dissolve 80 mg silver acetate (code 85140; Fluka, Buchs, Switzerland) in 40 ml of glass double-distilled water. Silver acetate crystals can be dissolved by continuous stirring within about 15 min.

(b) *Citrate buffer.* Dissolve 23.5 g of trisodium citrate dihydrate and 25.5 g citric acid monohydrate in 850 ml of deionized or distilled water. Prepare this buffer at least one day before use. It can be kept at 4°C for at least 2–3 weeks. Before use (at least at the day of use), adjust to pH 3.8 with citric acid solution.

(c) *Solution B.* Dissolve 200 mg hydroquinone in 40 ml citrate buffer.

(d) Just before use, mix solution A with solution B.

(e) *Silver amplification.* Place the slides vertically in a glass container (preferably with about 80 ml volume) and cover them by the mixture of solutions A and B. Staining intensity may be checked in the light microscope during the amplification process, which usually takes about 5 to 20 min, depending on incubation conditions and the amount of accessible nucleic acid target. In order to avoid overstaining, not too many sections at once should be developed. Stop development by washing slides in distilled water.

(f) Rinse the slides carefully in tap water for at least 5 min. After silver enhancement, sections can be counterstained with haematoxylin and eosin or nuclear Fast Red, dehydrated, and mounted.

Protocol 2.   DNA *in situ* hybridization with catalysed reporter deposition (CARD) using biotinylated tyramide and streptavidin–Nanogold

Practical considerations. This DNA detecting method can give superb sensitivity for DNA and has been tested using biotinylated cDNA probes as well as FITC-conjugated riboprobes. Its investigation with oligoprobes has not yet been completed. The technique was originally developed by us on cytospin preparations of cytological material containing only one to two copies of HPV

16. Using SiHa cells either spun on to glass slides or formalin-fixed, paraffin-embedded, sectioned, and mounted on glass slides, we were able to show that in the above system a real single gene copy sensitivity is obtained (Hacker *et al*. 1997; Zehbe *et al*. 1997). Because it is a method with the highest possible sensitivity, special precautions have to be taken into account. These include the use of freshly cut sections (not older than a few days) mounted on silanized (APES-coated) glass slides baked at 60°C on to the slide for 1 h, and changing or thoroughly cleaning the microtome knife for each new paraffin block. Tissues fixed in precipitating fixatives that contain heavy metals must first be deparaffinized and rehydrated and the trace metal content removed by Lugol's solution, followed by brief exposure to sodium thiosulfate; sections should be washed in PBS prior to proteinase K digestion. The Lugol's treatment should occur immediately prior to proteinase K and methanolic hydrogen peroxide treatment of the sections. Cytocentrifuge preparations can be used with the following procedure, but steps 1 and 2 should be eliminated (start at step 3). Cytospins should be air-dried prior to fixation in either neutral-buffered formalin or absolute ethanol. Buffers are as given in *Protocol 1*.

1. Deparaffinize formaldehyde-fixed sections in fresh xylene (2 × 15 min each).

2. Rinse in absolute ethanol (2 × 5 min each).

3. Treat with 3% H_2O_2 in methanol at RT for 30 min.

4. Rinse in double-distilled (ultrapure) water for 10 sec and then in PBS for 3 min.

5. Incubate sections with 0.01% proteinase K (code 1 373 196, stock solution of 18.6 mg/ml, from Boehringer Mannheim, Germany) in PBS at 37°C for 4–8 min, Duration has to be tested carefully, depending on tissue, fixation, and other factors. This treatment may partly destroy tissue morphology; however, it is necessary to open up binding sites for the probe to reach full sensitivity.

6. Rinse in 2 changes of PBS, 3 min each, then double distilled water for 10 sec, and dehydrate with graded alcohols (50% ethanol for 5 min, 70% ethanol for 5 min, and 98% ethanol 2 × 5 min each), and air dry the sections.

7. Prehybridize with 50% deionized formamide and 10% dextran sulfate in 2 × SSC buffer at 50°C for 5 min.

8. Carefully shake off the excess prehybridization block.

9. Add one drop of biotin- or FITC-conjugated DNA probe on to the section and cover with coverslip. Avoid air bubbles.

10. Heat sections on a heating block for denaturation of DNA (92–94°C) for 10 min.

11. Incubate the sections in a moist chamber at 37°C overnight or for 2 h.

12. Post-hybridization washes: 2 × SSC at 37 °C for 5 min, 0.5 × SSC at RT for 5 min, and then 0.2 × SSC at RT for 5 min.

13. Put the slides into Lugol's iodine solution, 5 min.

14. Wash in tap water and then double-distilled water.

15. Put into 2.5% sodium thiosulfate, until they are colourless (usually a few sec). Then wash in distilled water for 2 min.

16. Incubate with blocking solution at 37 °C for 30 min. Blocking solution is 4 × SSC containing 5% casein sodium salt (code C 8654, 9005-46-3; Sigma-Aldrich, Steinheim, Germany) or 0.5% blocking powder (NEN, as contained in the TSA-kit).

17. Brief wash in 4 × SSC containing 0.05% Tween-20)code no. 1332 465, Boehringer Mannheim).

18. Incubate with streptavidin–biotin–peroxidase complex (.e.g from Dako duett kit, Dako, Glostrup, Denmark) at RT for 30 min. The complex is dissolved in the above blocking solution at a concentration of 1:200.

19. Wash with 4 × SSC containing 0.05% Tween-20 (Boehringer Mannheim) 3 × for 5 min each, followed by PBS 2 × for 5 min each.

20. Incubate the sections with biotinylated tyramide (BT) (NEN) at RT for exactly 10 min. A stock solution of BT is prepared by adding 100 ml ethanol to the lyophilized reagent and is diluted 1:50 with the supplied amplification diluent as described in NEN's TSA kits mixed with distilled water at 1:1. According to the guidelines supplied with the kit, the working solution should contain 0.001 mg of BT per ml diluent, consisting of 0.2 M Tris–HCl, 10 mM imidazole, pH 8.8, and 0.01% H_2O_2.

21. Four consecutive washes in PBS containing 0.05% Tween-20 and 20% DMSO (dimethyl sulfoxide) at RT for 3 min each.

22. Immerse in PBS (pH 7.6) containing 0.1% fish–gelatin (45% concentrate—code no. G-7765—available from Sigma, Steinheim, Germany) (PBS–gelatin) for 5 min.

23. Incubate the sections with streptavidin–Nanogold (Nanoprobes, Stony Brook, USA) diluted 1:1500 in PBS pH 7.4 containing 1% BSA at RT for 60 min.

24. Wash in PBS pH 7.6, 2 × 5 min each.

25. Wash in PBS–gelatin pH 7.6 for 5 min.

26. Repeatedly wash in distilled water for at least 10 min altogether, the last 2 rinses in ultrapure water (EM grade).

27. Perform silver acetate autometallography (see addendum for Protocol 1).

28. When optimum staining is reached, immediately stop by rinsing carefully

in distilled or tap water for at least 3 min. Avoid post-fixation in sodium thiosulfate or photographic fixer for CARD ISH! After silver amplification, sections can be counterstained with haemotoxylin and eosin and/or nuclear Fast Red, dehydrated, and mounted in Permount™ or in DPX™ (BDH Chemicals, UK). Avoid the use of Eukitt.

Protocol 3.   RNA in situ hybridization with catalysed reporter deposition (CARD) using biotinylated tyramide and streptavidin–Nanogold

Practical considerations. The same precautions as given in Protocol 2 have to be taken. Because Protocol 3 gives the working procedure for RNA, additional hints are necessary. RNA is extremely labile and especially susceptible to destruction by RNase. RNA loss from tissue may occur owing to delays in primary fixation or the production of endonucleases by bacteria contaminating water baths and other equipment used in preparing tissue sections. There is little that the molecular pathologist can do to control fixation conditions beyond admonition of his or her colleagues and attention to processing protocols. Great care should be exercised to keep microtome blades and water baths cleaned and free of bacterial contamination, and sterile water should be used at least through the hybridization step. Either riboprobes or synthetic oligonucleotides coated with a reporter molecule such as FITC, digoxigenin, or biotin may be used. Hybridization conditions and nucleotide content must be appropriate for RNA rather than DNA hybridization. This protocol (given here for FITC as the reporter molecule) was developed for formalin-fixed tissue sections mounted on silanized glass slides. Tissues fixed in precipitating fixatives that contain heavy metals must first be deparaffinized and rehydrated and the trace metal content removed by Lugol's solution followed by brief exposure to sodium thiosulfate. This step should occur immediately prior to proteinase K and methanolic hydrogen peroxide treatment of the sections, and should be preceded by a 5 min wash in working PBS. Cytocentrifuge preparations can be used with the following procedure, but steps 1 and 2 should be eliminated (start at step 3). Cytospins should be air-dried prior to fixation in either neutral buffered formalin or absolute ethanol. Buffers are as given in Protocol 1.

1. Deparaffinize formaldehyde-fixed sections in fresh xylene (2 × 15 min each).

2. Rinse in absolute ethanol (2 × 5 min each).

3. Treat with 3% H_2O_2 in methanol at RT for 30 min.

4. Rinse in double-distilled (ultrapure) water for 10 sec and then in PBS for 3 min.

5. Incubate sections with 0.01% proteinase K (code 1 373 196, stock solution of 18.6 mg/ml, from Boehringer Mannheim, Germany) in PBS at 37°C for 4–8 min. Duration is critical and has to be tested carefully, depending on tissue, fixation, and other factors. This treatment may partly destroy tissue morphology; however, it is necessary to open-up binding sites for the probe to reach full sensitivity.

6. Rinse in 2 changes of PBS, 3 min each, then double-distilled water for 10 sec, and dehydrate with graded alcohols (50% ethanol for 5 min, 70% ethanol for 5 min, and 98% ethanol 2 × 5 min each) and air dry the sections.

7. Prehybridize with 50% deionized formamide and 10% dextran sulfate in 2 × SSC buffer at 50°C for 5 min.

8. Carefully shake off the excess prehybridization block.

9. Add one drop of FITC haptenated ribonucleotide or antisense oligo-nucleotide on the section and cover with coverslip. Avoid air bubbles.

10. Hybridize in a moist chamber at 37 °C overnight or for 2 h.

11. Post-hybridization washes: 2 × SSC at 37 °C for 5 min, 0.5 × SSC at RT for 5 min, and then 0.2 × SSC at RT for 5 min.

12. Wash in PBS for 3 min.

13. Incubate with mouse monoclonal anti-FITC (code no. BA-9200, Boehringer Mannheim) diluted in PBS at a working dilution of 1:1000 at RT for 30 min.

14. Wash in PBS twice for 3 min each.

15. Incubate sections with biotinylated goat anti-mouse IgG (Vector, Burlingame, USA) diluted in PBS at a working dilution of 1:200 at RT for 30 min.

16. Wash in PBS twice for 3 min each.

17. Put the slides into Lugol's iodine solution, 5 min.

18. Wash in tap water and then double-distilled water.

19. Put into 2.5% sodium thiosulfate, until they are colourless (usually a few sec). Then wash in distilled water for 2 min.

20. Incubate with blocking solution at 3°C for 30 min. Blocking solution is 4 × SSC containing 5% casein sodium salt (code C8654, 9005-46-3; Sigma-Aldrich, Steinheim, Germany) or 0.5% blocking powder (NEN, as contained in the TSA-kit).

21. Brief wash in 4 × SSC containing 0.05% Tween-20 (Boehringer Mannheim).

22. Incubate with streptavidin–biotin–peroxidase complex (.e.g from Dako duett kit) at RT for 30 min. The complex is dissolved in the above blocking solution at a concentration of 1:200.

23. Wash with 4 × SSC containing 0.05% Tween-20 (Boehringer Mannheim) 3 × for 5 min each, followed by PBS for 2 × for 5 min each.

24. Incubate the sections with biotinylated tyramide (BT) (NEN) at RT for exactly 10 min. A stock solution of BT is prepared by adding 100 ml ethanol to the lyophilized reagent and is diluted 1:50 with the supplied amplification diluent as described in NEN's TSA kits mixed with distilled water at 1:1. According to the guidelines supplied with the kit, the working solution should contain 0.001 mg of BT per ml diluent, consisting of 0.2 M Tris–HCl, 10 mM imidazole, pH 8.8 and 0.01% H_2O_2.

25. Four consecutive washes in PBS containing 0.05% Tween-20 and 20% DMSO (dimethyl sulfoxide) at RT for 3 min each.

26. Immerse in PBS (pH 7.6) containing 0.1% fish–gelatin (45% concentrate—code no. G-7765—available from Sigma, Steinheim, Germany) (PBS–gelatin) for 5 min.

27. Incubate the sections with streptavidin–Nanogold (Nanoprobes, Stony Brook, NY, USA) diluted 1:1500 in PBS pH 7.4 containing 1% BSA at RT for 60 min.

28. Wash in PBS pH 7.6 2 × 5 min each.

29. Wash in PBS–gelatin pH 7.6 for 5 min.

30. Repeatedly wash in distilled water for at least 10 min altogether, the last 2 rinses in ultrapure water (EM grade).

31. Perform silver acetate autometallography (see addendum in Protocol 1).

32. When optimum staining is reached, immediately stop by rinsing carefully in distilled or tap water for at least 3 min. Avoid post-fixation in sodium thiosulfate or photographic fixer for CARD ISH! After silver amplification, sections can be counterstained with haematoxylin and eosin and/or nuclear Fast Red, dehydrated, and mounted in Permount™ or in DPX™ (BDH Chemicals, UK). Avoid the use of Eukitt.

Index

List of suppliers

Amersham

Amersham International plc., Lincoln Place, Green End, Aylesbury, Buckinghamshire HP20 2TP, UK.

Amersham Corporation, 2636 South Clearbrook Drive, Arlington Heights, IL 60005, USA.

Anderman

Anderman and Co. Ltd., 145 London Road, Kingston-Upon-Thames, Surrey KT17 7NH, UK.

ATCC (American Type Culture Collection), 10801 University Boulevard, Manassas, VA 20110–2209, USA.

BDH, Merk Ltd., Poole, Dorset, UK.

Beckman Instruments

Beckman Instruments UK Ltd., Progress Road, Sands Industrial Estate, High Wycombe, Buckinghamshire HP12 4JL, UK.

Beckman Instruments Inc., PO Box 3100, 2500 Harbor Boulevard, Fullerton, CA 92634, USA.

Becton Dickinson

Becton Dickinson and Co., Between Towns Road, Cowley, Oxford OX4 3LY, UK.

Becton Dickinson and Co., 2 Bridgewater Lane, Lincoln Park, NJ 07035, USA.

Bio

Bio 101 Inc., c/o Statech Scientific Ltd, 61–63 Dudley Street, Luton, Bedfordshire LU2 0HP, UK.

Bio 101 Inc., PO Box 2284, La Jolla, CA 92038–2284, USA.

Bio-Rad Laboratories

Bio-Rad Laboratories Ltd., Bio-Rad House, Maylands Avenue, Hemel Hempstead HP2 7TD, UK.

Bio-Rad Laboratories, Division Headquarters, 3300 Regatta Boulevard, Richmond, CA 94804, USA.

Boehringer Mannheim

Boehringer Mannheim UK (Diagnostics and Biochemicals) Ltd., Bell Lane, Lewes, East Sussex BN17 1LG, UK.

Boehringer Mannheim Corporation, Biochemical Products, 9115 Hague Road, P.O. Box 504 Indianopolis, IN 46250–0414, USA.

Boehringer Mannheim Biochemica, GmbH, Sandhofer Str. 116, Postfach 310120 D-6800 Ma 31, Germany.

British Drug Houses (BDH) Ltd., Poole, Dorset UK.

Cambio, 34 Newnham Road, Cambridge, CB3 9EY, UK.

Difco Laboratories
Difco Laboratories Ltd., P.O. Box 14B, Central Avenue, West Molesey, Surrey KT8 2SE, UK.
Difco Laboratories, P.O. Box 221058, Detroit, MI 48232–7058, USA.
Du Pont
Dupont (UK) Ltd., Industrial Products Division, Wedgwood Way, Stevenage, Herts, SH1 4Q, UK.
Du Pont Co. (Biotechnology Systems Division), P.O. Box 80024, Wilmington, DE 19880–002, USA.
European Collection of Animal Cell Culture, Division of Biologics, PHLS Centre for Applied Microbiology and Research, Porton Down, Salisbury, Wilts. SP4 0JG, UK.
Falcon (Falcon is a registered trademark of Becton Dickinson and Co.)
Fisher Scientific Co., 711 Forbest Avenue, Pittsburgh, PA 15219–4785, USA.
Flow Laboratories, Woodcock Hill, Harefield Road, Rickmansworth, Herts. WD3 1PQ, UK.
Fluka
Fluka-Chemie AG, CH-9470, Buchs, Switzerland.
Fluka Chemicals Ltd., The Old Brickyard, New Road, Gillingham, Dorset SP8 4JL, UK.
Gibco BRL
Gibco BRL (Life Technologies Ltd.), Trident House, Renfrew Road, Paisley PA3 4EF, UK.
Gibco BRL (Life Technologies Inc.), 3175 Staler Road, Grand Island, NY 14072–0068, USA.
Arnold R. Horwell, 73 Maygrove Road, West Hampstead, London NW6 2BP, UK.
Hybaid
Hybaid Ltd., 111–113 Waldegrave Road, Teddington, Middlesex TW11 8LL, UK.
Hybaid, National Labnet Corporation, P.O. Box 841, Woodbridge, N.J. 07095, USA.
HyClone Laboratories 1725 South HyClone Road, Logan,UT 84321, USA.
International Biotechnologies Inc., 25 Science Park, New Haven, Connecticut 06535, USA.
Imagenetics, Home Automation, Security, Entertainment, 7000 Terminal Square, Upper Darby, PA19082, USA.
Invitrogen Corporation
Invitrogen Corporation 3985 B Sorrenton Valley Building, San Diego, C.A. 92121, USA.
Invitrogen Corporation c/o British Biotechnology Products Ltd., 4–10 The Quadrant, Barton Lane, Abingdon, OX14 3YS, UK.
Kodak: Eastman Fine Chemicals 343 State Street, Rochester, NY, USA.

Life Technologies Inc., 8451 Helgerman Court, Gaithersburg, MN 20877, USA.

Merck

Merck Industries Inc., 5 Skyline Drive, Nawthorne, NY 10532, USA.

Merck, Frankfurter Strasse, 250, Postfach 4119, D-64293, Germany.

Millipore

Millipore (UK) Ltd., The Boulevard, Blackmoor Lane, Watford, Herts WD1 8YW, UK.

Millipore Corp./Biosearch, P.O. Box 255, 80 Ashby Road, Bedford, MA 01730, USA.

Nano Pobes, Stony Brook, New York, USA.

NEN (New England Nuclear), Life Science Products, Boston, Massachusetts, USA.

New England Biolabs (NBL)

New England Biolabs (NBL), 32 Tozer Road, Beverley, MA 01915–5510, USA.

New England Biolabs (NBL), c/o CP Labs Ltd., P.O. Box 22, Bishops Stortford, Herts CM23 3 DH. UK.

Nikon Corporation, Fuji Building, 2–3 Marunouchi 3-chome, Chiyoda-ku, Tokyo, Japan.

ONCOR, 209 Perry Parkway, Gaithersburg, MD 20877, USA.

Perkin-Elmer

Perkin-Elmer Ltd., Maxwell Road, Beaconsfield, Bucks. HP9 1QA, UK.

Perkin Elmer Ltd., Post Office Lane, Beaconsfield, Bucks. HP9 1QA, UK.

Perkin Elmer-Cetus (The Perkin-Elmer Corporation), 761 Main Avenue, Norwalk, CT 0689, USA.

Pharmacia Biotech Europe Procordia EuroCentre, Rue de laa Fuse-e 62, B-1130 Brussels, Belgium.

Parmacia Biosystems

Pharmacia Biosystems Ltd., (Biotechnology Division), Davy Avenue, Knowlhill, Milton Keynes MK5 8PH, UK.

Pharmacia LKB Biotechnology AB, Björngatan 30, S-75182 Uppsala, Sweden.

Promega

Promega Ltd., Delta House, Enterprise Road, Chilworth Research Centre, Southampton, UK.

Promega Corporation, 2800 Woods Hollow Road, Madison, WI 53711–5399, USA.

Qiagen

Qiagen Inc., c/o Hybaid, 111–113 Waldegrave Road, Teddington, Middlesex, TW11 8LL, UK.

Qiagen Inc., 9259 Eton Avenue, Chatsworth, C.A. 91311, USA.

Schleicher and Schuell

Schleicher and Schuell Inc., Keene, NH 03431A, USA.

Schleicher and Schuell Inc., D-3354 Dassel, Germany, Schleicher and Schuell Inc., c/o Andermann and Company Ltd.

Shandon Scientific Ltd., Chadwick Road, Astmoore, Runcorn, Cheshire WA7 1PR, UK.

Sigma Chemical Company

Sigma Chemical Company (UK), Fancy Road, Poole, Dorset BH17 7NH, UK.

Sigma Chemical Company, 3050 Spruce Street, P.O. Box 14508, St. Louis, MO 63178–9916.

Sorvall DuPont Company, Biotechnology Division, P.O. Box 80022, Wilmington, DE 19880–0022, USA.

Stratagene

Strategene Ltd., Unit 140, Cambridge Innovation Centre, Milton Road, Cambridge CB4 4FG, UK.

Strategene Inc., 11011 North Torrey Pines Road, La Jolla, CA 92037, USA.

United States Biochemical, P.O. Box 22400, Cleveland, OH 44122, USA.

Vector Laboratories, Burlington California, CA94010, USA.

Wellcome Reagents, Langley Court, Beckenham, Kent BR3 3BS, UK.

Ingram Content Group UK Ltd.
Milton Keynes UK
UKHW020417150623
423418UK00004B/271